TIA as Acute Cerebrovascular Syndrome

Frontiers of Neurology and Neuroscience

Vol. 33

Series Editor

J. Bogousslavsky Montreux

TIA as Acute Cerebrovascular Syndrome

Volume Editors

S. Uchiyama Tokyo

P. Amarenco Paris

K. Minematsu Osaka

K.S.L. Wong Hong Kong

25 figures, 7 in color and 14 tables, 2014

KARGER Basel · Freiburg · Paris · London · New York · New Delhi · Bangkok · Beijing · Tokyo · Kuala Lumpur · Singapore · Sydney

Frontiers of Neurology and Neuroscience
Vols. 1–18 were published as Monographs in Clinical Neuroscience

Shinichiro Uchiyama
Tokyo Women's Medical University School of Medicine
Department of Neurology
Tokyo 162-8666
Japan

Kazuo Minematsu
Cerebrovascular Division
Department of Medicine
National Cerebral and Cardiovascular Center
Suita, Osaka 565-8565
Japan

Pierre Amarenco
Department of Neurology and Stroke Centre
AP-HP, Bichat-Claude Bernard Hospital
University Paris Diderot
Sorbonne Paris Cité, INSERM U698
FR–75018 Paris
France

K.S. Lawrence Wong
Chinese University of Hong Kong
Prince of Wales Hospital
Department of Medicine & Therapeutics
Hong Kong
Hong Kong

Library of Congress Cataloging-in-Publication Data

TIA as acute cerebrovascular syndrome / volume editors, S. Uchiyama, P. Amarenco, K. Minematsu, K.S.L. Wong.
p. ; cm. -- (Frontiers of neurology and neuroscience, ISSN 1660-4431 ; Vol. 33)
Includes bibliographical references and index.
ISBN 978-3-318-02458-6 (hard cover : alk. paper) -- ISBN 978-3-318-02459-3 (electronic version)
I. Uchiyama, Shin'ichiro, editor of compilation. II. Amarenco, Pierre, editor of compilation. III. Minematsu, Kazuo, editor of compilation. IV. Wong, K. S. Lawrence, editor of compilation. V. Series: Frontiers of neurology and neuroscience ; v. 33. 1660-4431
[DNLM: 1. Ischemic Attack, Transient--therapy. W1 MO568C v.33 2014 / WL 356]
RC388.5
616.8'1--dc23
2013031979

Bibliographic Indices. This publication is listed in bibliographic services, including Current Contents® and Index Medicus.

Disclaimer. The statements, opinions and data contained in this publication are solely those of the individual authors and contributors and not of the publisher and the editor(s). The appearance of advertisements in the book is not a warranty, endorsement, or approval of the products or services advertised or of their effectiveness, quality or safety. The publisher and the editor(s) disclaim responsibility for any injury to persons or property resulting from any ideas, methods, instructions or products referred to in the content or advertisements.

Drug Dosage. The authors and the publisher have exerted every effort to ensure that drug selection and dosage set forth in this text are in accord with current recommendations and practice at the time of publication. However, in view of ongoing research, changes in government regulations, and the constant flow of information relating to drug therapy and drug reactions, the reader is urged to check the package insert for each drug for any change in indications and dosage and for added warnings and precautions. This is particularly important when the recommended agent is a new and/or infrequently employed drug.

www.karger.com
Printed in Germany on acid-free and non-aging paper (ISO 97069) by Kraft Druck, Ettlingen
ISSN 1660–4431
e-ISSN 1662–2804
ISBN 978–3–318–02458–6
e-ISBN 978–3–318–02459–3

Contents

Preface

Transient ischemic attack (TIA) is well known to be a prodromal syndrome of ischemic stroke. However, TIA is easily neglected or underestimated by patients or their families because the symptoms naturally disappear without any treatment. Even by general physicians, TIA is not prioritized since it is regarded as minor stroke. However, early after the onset of TIA, patients are at very high risk of stroke.

There is no global consensus on the definition of TIA. In the classical criteria, TIA is defined as focal neurologic brain or retinal ischemic symptoms which disappear within 24 h. However, the TIA Working Group in the United States defined TIA as brain or retinal ischemic symptoms within 1 h of the duration without responsible ischemic lesions. Afterwards, the American Heart Association and the American Stroke Association redefined TIA as transient focal ischemic symptoms in the brain, retina, or spinal cord without evidence of ischemic lesion regardless of the duration of symptoms.

On the other hand, the distribution of the duration of TIA with positive MRI diffusion-weighted image is continuous without any specific cutoff point. Thus, it is not possible to differentiate TIA from ischemic stroke only by the duration of symptoms. Therefore, there would be no meaning in differentiating TIA from acute ischemic stroke (AIS) by the duration of symptoms in acute settings. Rather, TIA and AIS should be recognized on the same spectrum of acute ischemic syndrome in the central nervous system.

In the Steering Committee of TIAregistry.org, which is an investigator-driven, international, multicenter cooperative, observational study of TIA and minor AIS, we proposed a new concept termed acute cerebrovascular syndrome (ACVS), which includes TIA in acute settings and AIS. The concept of ACVS is comparable to acute coronary syndrome (ACS), which includes unstable angina and acute myocardial infarction. However, unlike ACS, the mechanism of ACVS is complicated, including not only large artery atherosclerosis similar to ACS but also cardioembolism or small vessel occlusion. In addition, there are no measurable biomarkers for ACVS such as troponins for ACS. Nevertheless, the concept of ACVS is practical to emphasize the importance of immediate evaluation and starting treatment to prevent subsequent stroke in patients with acute settings of TIA. Therefore, TIA in acute settings as well as AIS should be recognized as ACVS, which is a medical emergency.

In patients with TIA in acute settings, after immediate examination, antithrombotic therapy as well as risk factor management with antihypertensives, statins, and glucose-lowering drugs are promptly required. As to antithrombotic therapy, dual antiplatelet therapy may be effective to prevent early stroke recurrence in patients with non-cardioembolic TIA for aggressive inhibition of platelet activation, while novel oral anticoagulants for rapid inhibition of coagulation activation may be useful for preventing early stroke recurrence in patients with cardioembolic TIA due to atrial fibrillation. In patients with severe arterial stenosis and resistant to medical treatment, surgical or intravascular intervention with carotid endarterectomy or carotid artery stenting as an emergency procedure may be necessitated.

TIA clinics may be very useful for immediate evaluation and management of acute TIA patients. They accept TIA patients 24 h a day, 365 days a year. In reality, TIA clinic was reported to be very effective in reducing risk of stroke during 90 days after TIA. The report showed that this effect was brought about by early starting of dual antiplatelet therapy, statin use, and single or dual antihypertensive treatment.

In the field of cardiology, the terminology of ACS including unstable angina and acute myocardial infarction was used for the campaign to save lives from cardiac death, which was very successful for reducing the overall death rate. In the field of neurology, terminology of ACVS is expected to be helpful in remarkably reducing early subsequent risk of stroke, which is the leading cause of death and disability worldwide.

This book covers all topics of TIA as ACVS including the definition, concept, etiology, epidemiology, symptomatology, risk scores, neuroimaging, neurosonology, acute management, primary and secondary prevention, and guidelines. The authors of the excellent updated reviews in the respective chapters are all top opinion experts in stroke neurology. We hope many readers worldwide will find this book useful for clinical practice and research.

Shinichiro Uchiyama, Tokyo

Uchiyama S, Amarenco P, Minematsu K, Wong KSL (eds): TIA as Acute Cerebrovascular Syndrome.
Front Neurol Neurosci. Basel, Karger, 2014, vol 33, pp 1–10 (DOI: 10.1159/000351883)

History of Transient Ischemic Attack Definition

Jay P. Mohr

Doris & Stanley Tananbaum Stroke Center, Neurological Institute, Columbia University Medical Center, New York, N.Y., USA

Abstract

Transient ischemic attacks have been recognized as a clinical entity for well over a century. Efforts before the availability of modern imaging to establish a diagnosis of inferred ischemic stroke led to acceptance of too long a time period (>24 h) compared with the actual typical events lasting <24 min (usually 5–15 min). Revision of the time period has improved diagnostic yield and discovered many whose image-documented acute infarct is associated with a short clinical course.

As of January 2013, PubMed contains close to 20,000 references in which transient ischemic attack – also known as TIA – is cited in the title or keywords. This large a number suggests the subject has become one of the many acronyms in clinical medicine, its definition and application familiar to all. Sadly, not entirely so.

As a starting point, the ICD-9 code, in common use, for code 435 'transient cerebral ischemia' (no mention of attacks) is notable to its lack of detail. No mention is made of time, the mechanism is inferred to be '...vascular insufficiency' and excludes that most ambiguous of diagnoses, 'acute cerebrovascular insufficiency NOS [not otherwise stated]'. Little wonder those entering the neurovascular field are unclear on the setting where the term TIA can be applied (table 1).

There are rare references to intermittent symptoms discovered at autopsy due to infarction dating well back past the prior century [1]. (Limits of reference numbers for this chapter preclude many citations, leaving the author to the use of examples.)

Table 1. Various sets of terms used to describe TIA in ICD-9 coding

435 Transient cerebral ischemia
Includes Cerebrovascular insufficiency (acute) with transient focal neurological signs and symptoms Insufficiency of basilar, carotid, and vertebral arteries Spasm of cerebral arteries
Excludes Acute cerebrovascular insufficiency NOS (437.1) That due to any condition classifiable to 433 (433.0–433.9)

'Attack'

Working backwards through the elements, the term, 'attack', suggests something sudden. The published experience emphasizes a change from normal, but none of the current definitions clarifies whether the event reaches its peak of neurological features immediately, or the means by which the syndrome fades to normal.

The best characterized have been those affecting vision in one eye. Published reports and the author's experience with patients have – in the vast majority – cited a shade falling smoothly over vision, some completely to the bottom, some stopping – usually midway. The loss of vision is usually described as blank, rarely black. Although the term 'curtain' has been used, the term usually refers to the modern theatrical straight-across curtain falling from above, not the classical curtain which lifts from the center to the upper corners of both side. The author has found no examples of a 'shade' which appears to move to or from the side as in a sliding door. Fortification features have not been described. One remarkable report cited recurrent sectoranopia abnormalities and was traced to a stenosis of a retinal branch [2]. Fisher's famous case, published in 1959 [3] required approximately 45 min for the white plug to work its way distally and disappear, vision improving in the wake of the clearing. His attempts to explain the mechanism have left some authors citing embolism, others perfusion failure from high-grade stenosis in a feeding vessel.

For hemispheral or brainstem syndromes, most clinicians have heard from patients of a premonitory general sense of unease, some vaguely aware something was in the offing but undefined until the focal features appeared, some hours, others over a day or more later. (The delay in symptomatic onset has been amply demonstrated by many unpublished cases where an aberrant embolus during a catheter procedure generated angiographic evidence of the embolus, but the focal neurological event was delayed minutes to hours later. Such delays challenge common assumptions that the symptomatic onset coincides with the time of occlusion.)

The reported focal features have also shown intensification in either quantitative (e.g. more weakness) or qualitative (e.g. weakness then also numbness) degree, some-

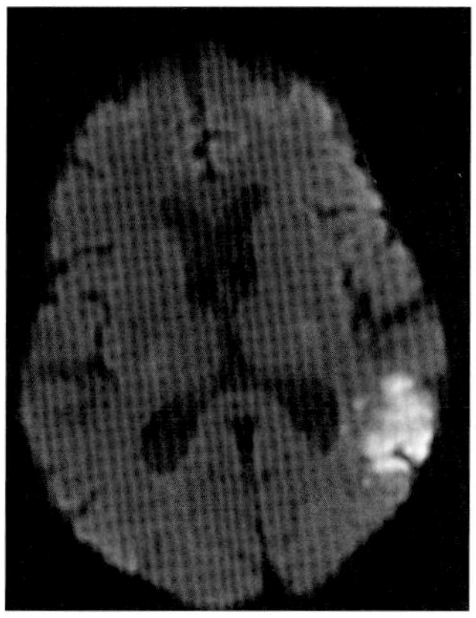

Fig. 1. Symptomatic focal DWI-positive infarct with syndrome lasting 10 min.

times both occurring in the same attack [4]. Convexity TIA and stroke may feature pseudo-median or pseudo-ulnar syndromes [5]. Isolated mutism [6] or sensory aphasia are unusual, but a recent case seen by the author suffered mutism for <10 min; seen at the end of the time period by a group of experienced neurologists, he passed for normal on examination, busily working with his wife to pay monthly bills while hospitalized for cardiac disease. A focal DWI-positive infarct was found just posterior to the superior temporal plane (see fig. 1).

Little wonder many can be diagnosed as migraine aurae. No definition yet accounts for these variables, as the main emphasis is on the inferred ischemic nature and duration. The current ICD9 code for diagnosis leaves the features of the clinical syndrome up to the clinician to decide.

'Ischemic'

That such attacks are by definition 'ischemic' has been challenged by many critics, who point to the brief migraine aura, non-convulsive epilepsy, even a few examples of small parenchymatous hemorrhage with subsidence of the symptoms. There is also ample literature to demonstrate the ischemic symptoms may experience rapid improvement (within hours) despite documentation of clinically correlated focal brain infarction. Further, examples have been published of a susceptibility of symptomatic relapse from exposure to benzodiazepines administered up to a week after disappearance of symptoms and brain imaging showing no DWI-positive foci [7].

Brief events have also been described from a large variety of ischemic causes, among them paroxysmal atrial fibrillation, bacterial endocarditis, thrombotic thrombocytopenic purpura, arterial dissections, minor embolism via patent cardiac foramen ovale, even the first stage of ruptured aneurysm [8].

'Transient'

Even the time frame suggested by term 'transient' has been a subject of a wide spectrum of definitions. The modern history dates from 1954 at the second Princeton Conference (all the biannual conferences were held at the Nassau Inn in Princeton, NJ, until the conference began its peripatetic movements in 1980).

The first, held under the auspices of the American Heart Association, with NY Hospital/Cornell Cardiologist Dr. Irving S. Wright as chairman, and Cornell Internist E. Hugh Luckey, as editor, was simply titled 'Cerebral Vascular Diseases'. It was attended by many of the small cadre of leading neurologists of the time, including R.D. Adams and C.M. Fisher (Massachusetts General Hospital, Boston), J.M. Foley (then at Boston City Hospital), H.H. Merritt (Neurological Institute, New York), C.H. Millikan (Mayo, Rochester, Minn., USA). Dr. Ellen McDevitt (also of Cornell) presented results of treatment of valvular heart disease and atrial fibrillation with warfarin.

The second conference, in 1956, the number of attendees much larger, included R.G. Siekert (Mayo, Rochester, Minn., USA), W.R. Brain (Maida Vale, London, UK), E.A. Gurdjian (Wayne State, Detroit, Mich., USA), A. Heyman (Duke, Durham, N.C., USA), J.S. Meyer (Baylor, Houston, Tex., USA), P. Scheinberg (U Miami), and J.P. Whisnant (Mayo, Rochester, Minn., USA). C.M. Fisher made an oral presentation titled 'Intermittent cerebral ischemia'. In it, he provided an extensive characterization of 'transient ischemic attacks' which he noted '…may last from a few seconds up to several hours, the most common duration being a few seconds up to 5 or 10 min'. The published report of the discussion shows no disagreements with this definition, or the brief time frame, in the published report of discussion afterwards [9].

Sufficient interest in the subject led to a publication in an issue of *Neurology* (the journal *Stroke* still in utero) titled 'A classification of and outline of cerebrovascular diseases' [10]. The authors included many who had attended the conference. Included in the definitions was one for 'cerebral infarction', which noted 'The neurologic deficit may be maximal when first discovered or may require several hours or even a day or so to evolve'. (All this text was generated by authors whose experience was based on clinical evaluation, most of whom had had some training in neuropathology. Tissue imaging by the likes of CT and MR was decades in their future.)

By 1961 when the 3rd Princeton Conference was held, interest in the time-based definitions for stroke had progressed to a 'TIA Working Group' led by J.F. Toole (Bowman Gray, Winston Salem, N.C., USA). R.G. Siekert, attending his third Princeton Conference, offered a definition of three stages of focal arterial disease, the last being 'completed stroke', describing 'a focal neurologic deficit, which is *stable for hours or days* and then tends to decrease in amount'. At the same conference, C.M. Fisher presented findings on anticoagulant therapy from the National Cooperative Study begun in 1958. Fisher offered the view 'transient ischemic attacks (T.I.A.)…. refers to the occurrence of single or multiple episodes of cerebral dysfunction *lasting no longer than one hour* and clearing without significant residuum' [11].

As before, no specific time frame was provided for diagnoses of ischemic stroke attributed to thrombosis and suspected thrombosis or embolism. In a later chapter in the conference proceedings, R.N. Baker refers to most of his cases of 'completed' strokes as having 'been *stable for more than 48 h*' [12].

Despite these publications, the literature failed to reflect much impact on the time frame. The only reference found by the present author for duration was that of Acheson and Hutchinson. In their 1964 article titled 'Observations on the natural history of transient cerebral ischaemia' they note that that attacks '...should be less than one hour' [13].

Also in 1964, John Marshall, then the leading neurologist for stroke in the UK (cited by one retired French neurologist as 'then the sheriff in these parts') published a single-author review in the *Quarterly Journal of Medicine* entitled 'The natural history of transient ischaemic attacks' [14]. The case material cited 75 cases as lasting 'minutes', 17 '30 min', 13 '1 h', and 38 'several hours'. (No definition was given for 'several'.) He defined transient ischemic attacks as:

> 'A disturbance of neurological function of less than 24 h' duration occurring in the territory of supply of the carotid or vertebrobasilar arteries...' ... '...the typical T.I.A. is an attack of only brief duration, usually lasting less than five minutes. More prolonged attacks, however, do occur, and although transient is perhaps a misnomer, they do share the characteristic of leaving little or no residual deficit. The same can, of course, be said of a small percentage of major strokes; hence some arbitrary time limit has to be set.'

He made no reference to earlier proposal of TIA as brief as 5–10 min. After an interval of 14 years, in 1977 he and co-authors M.J. Harrison and D.J. Thomas published in the *British Medical Journal* an article entitled 'Relevance of duration of transient ischaemic attacks in carotid territory' [15]. They cited 116 patients, separating them into group 1 (<1 h), group 2 (>1 h), and group 3 (both types). Those with angiographic findings of stenosis or atheroma were mainly in group 1. Independently, the same year M.S. Pessin, G.W. Duncan, J.P. Mohr and D. Poskanzer published an angiographic study of carotid TIA in 115 patients in the *New England Journal of Medicine* [16]. This work at the Massachusetts General Hospital was a substudy from the National Institute on Neurological Disease and Blindness (NINDB) cooperative project. Those with severe stenosis or occlusion had TIAs lasting 5–15 min; those with widely patent carotids had events lasting well beyond an hour.

No revision of the timetable appeared in any of the major statements of disease definitions even as late as 1975 [17].

In the mid-1980s, anticipating trials to intervene early in hopes of aborting developing ischemia [18], NINDS funded a contract to study the timing of appearance of abnormalities on CT scan and the then early MR scan. The two centers Columbia University and the University of Iowa were able to enroll 80 patients in a 180-min time frame [19]. Sixty-eight patients were recruited within 4 h, and an additional 12 patients within 24 h. Seventy-five strokes were due to infarction and five to hemorrhage. The median time to first scan was 132 min. Although some of the infarctions in 75 patients were detected within 1 h, the fraction of positive first scans approached an

Table 2. Time from event to DWI imaging, percentage positive or negative

Year	Study	n	DWI+	Hours	DWI–	DWI+
2004	Restrepo [21]	58	67%	<24	0.96	6.8
2002	Rovira [22]	58	67%	<24		

Table 3. Summary of the literature showing duration of events and percentage DWI+

Duration of symptoms	Total (n = 2,206)
>24 h CT/MR+	1,498 (67.9%)
>24 h CT/MR–	568 (25.7%)
<24 h CT/MR+	140 (6.3%)

asymptote at 2–3 h. There was a marginally significant correlation between early positive brain imaging and the severity of the stroke. Some patients had initially positive CT and/or MRI scans, but their neurological examination had returned to normal by 24 h. This study helped settle a 90-min window for acute ischemic imaging and indicated treatment outcomes could be improved by earlier treatment [20].

The following decades saw the widespread use and improved imaging by MR. The two publications cited in table 2 are among many examples showing a striking percentage of DWI-positive foci for patients imaged well within the 24-hour time frame. These publications clearly documented 24 h was too long to wait to decide if the acute syndrome was a stroke, but left unclear how many might experience syndrome remission. The clinical findings of these patients with absent imaging data *would have earlier been classified on clinical grounds alone* as a TIA.

As an example of the impact of modern imaging, the large Warfarin Aspirin Ischemic Stroke Study (WARSS) attempted to introduce the 1-hour definition, based on the CT/R study, but yielded to the <24 h given the wish to relate the findings to those of other trials (table 3). Yet, even in the WARSS the baseline data contained 6.3% whose initial CT or MR was positive for the event despite imaging done within 24 h [23].

Modern Redefinition

Alert to the ambiguities in the definitions, and wishing some improvement in definitions, Boehringer Ingelheim sponsored a series of meetings hoping to generate a modern definition. Held in several attractive resort sites, the participants worked up a series of presentations, which finally culminated in the proposal published in 2001 in the *New England Journal of Medicine* [24].

> We propose a new definition for TIA encompassing the concept that patients who experience a TIA will have no objective evidence of acute infarction in the affected brain region. Therefore, patients who have transient focal symptoms of brain ischemia – and upon diagnostic evaluation are found to have an acute brain infarction – would no longer be classified as having a TIA, regardless of the duration of clinical symptoms. With this new definition, the difference between a TIA and a stroke becomes similar to the distinction between an episode of angina pectoris and an MI. Angina is a symptom of cardiac ischemia, which is usually brief but may be prolonged, without MI. If there is objective evidence of myocardial damage, then the term 'MI' is applied.
>
> We propose the following redefinition for the term 'TIA':
>
> *A transient ischemic attack (TIA) is a brief episode of neurologic dysfunction caused by focal brain or retinal ischemia, with clinical symptoms typically lasting <1 h and without evidence of accompanying infarction.*
>
> The corollary is that permanent clinical signs or appropriate brain imaging abnormalities define cerebral infarction – that is, *stroke*. While preserving the TIA concept, this new definition abandons the arbitrary 24-hour limit and substitutes general parameters that more closely match the typical duration of TIAs. Furthermore, the specific exclusion of patients with acute brain infarction serves to more clearly distinguish a TIA from a stroke. This redefinition is more in keeping with the definitions used to describe myocardial ischemic events.
>
> A limitation to this concept is that patients who receive brain imaging studies for the evaluation of their TIAs may be classified differently than individuals who are not imaged. However, as neurodiagnostic procedures continue to advance, the proposed definition allows patients to be classified based on the best available data for the individual patient. In addition, the new definition avoids assigning an arbitrary time limit for the maximal duration of a TIA. For example, a patient with a 2-hour clinical episode that causes a small brain infarction would be classified as having a stroke rather than a TIA, while a patient with an identical episode and no evidence of acute infarction (either because no imaging was performed or imaging studies were negative) would be diagnosed with TIA.

Current Impact of the Modern TIA Definition

The impact of the 1 h rule on current schemes for diagnosis seems at best to have been minor. The current ICD9 coding document has no reference to timing.

There is ample modern evidence that confirms earlier impressions that TIA is a predictor of subsequent ischemic stroke, and that the time between TIA and stroke can be quite short: 8–10% during the 7 days after a TIA or minor stroke [25–27]. It is also clear that early intervention has a major effect on reducing the subsequent ischemic stroke risk [28].

Despite the steadily accumulating evidence, even the elegant and practical scoring systems recently devised to identify risk factors for stroke after TIA continue to use the 24 h rule [29, 30]. A similar reliance on the 'classical definition, a TIA was defined as an acute loss of focal cerebral or ocular function with symptoms lasting <24 h…' is found in a recent large 2-year study of efforts to diagnose the subsequent stroke using a variety of etiology classification [31].

In the nearly 5 decades since the initial efforts to define a time frame for TIA, clinical trials of ischemic stroke continued to use a <24 h definition when classifying events. The reason seems to have been the hesitation to introduce new definitions where the trial was intended to assess a given agent's effects as prophylaxis or reversal of an acute stroke syndrome.

In the current year (2013), the <24 h definition still applied to all seven of the articles cited in PubMed with transient ischemic attack in the title. Many of these articles were large national databases stretched over several years. One report [32] noted the reclassification of the event into stroke if imaging demonstrated an acute infarct; no data were presented for the frequency of this group.

None of these publications are criticized for their focus on outcomes, only for the difficulty assessing which of the events lasting <1 h prove to be the majority, or, more likely, remain among those disregarded as too brief to be important, too brief to create a sense of concern, and too brief be transported to a clinical setting for evaluation. The development of centers for acute evaluation of TIA is a welcome development, and can be hoped to expand insights into the fate for the brief attacks [33].

As a starting point, the ICD9 code for 'transient cerebral ischemia' (no mention of attacks) is notable for its lack of detail. No mention is made of time, the mechanism is inferred to be '...vascular insufficiency' and excludes that most ambiguous of diagnoses, 'acute cerebrovascular insufficiency NOS [not otherwise stated]. Little wonder those entering the neurovascular field are unclear on the setting where the term TIA can be applied.

The current 2013 ICD-10-CM Diagnosis Code G45.9, to be replaced in 2014, represents some progress:

> Transient cerebral ischemic attack, unspecified: recurring, transient episodes of neurologic dysfunction caused by cerebral ischemia; onset is usually sudden, often when the patient is active; the attack may last a few seconds to several hours; neurologic symptoms depend on the artery involved.
>
> A brief attack (from a few minutes to an hour) of cerebral dysfunction of vascular origin with no persistent neurological deficit.
>
> Applicable to:
> Spasm of cerebral artery
> TIA
> Transient cerebral ischemia NOS
> Transient cerebral ischemic attack, unspecified

It remains as C.M. Fisher proposed in 1956 and noted in his last publication (an editorial) that, at the least, a '...TIA sounds an alarm' [34].

References

1 Bramwell B: A remarkable case of aphasia. Brain 1898;21:343–373.

2 Wolpow ER, Lupton RG: Transient vertical monocular hemianopsia with anomalous retinal artery branching. Stroke 1981;12:691–692.

3 Fisher CM: Observations of the fundus oculi in transient monocular blindness. Neurology 1959;9:337.

4 Loeb C, Gandolfo C: Transient ischemic neurologic deficits; in Vinken PJ, Bruyn GW (eds): Handbook of Clinical Neurology. Amsterdam, Elsevier, 1988, vol 53, pp 257–290.

5 Timsit SG, Sacco RL, Mohr JP, Foulkes MA, Tatemichi TK, Wolf PA, Price TR, Hier DB: Early clinical differentiation of cerebral infarction from severe atherosclerotic stenosis and cardioembolism. Stroke 1992;23:486–491.

6 Mohr JP: Rapid amelioration of motor aphasia. Arch Neurol 1973;28:77–82.

7 Lazar RM, Fitzsimmons BF, Marshall RS, Mohr JP, Berman MF: Midazolam challenge reinduces neurological deficits after transient ischemic attack. Stroke 2003;34:794–796.

8 Mohr JP: Improving the assessment of TIAs. Eur J Neurol 2012;19:1.

9 Fisher CM: Intermittent cerebral ischemia; in Wright IS, Millikan CH (eds): Cerebral Vascular Disease. New York, Grune and Stratton, 1958, pp 81–97.

10 Ad Hoc Committee on Cerebrovascular Disease of the Advisory Council of the National Institute on Neurological Disease and Blindness: A classification of and outline of cerebrovascular diseases. Neurology 1958;8:395–434.

11 Toole JF: The Willis Lecture: transient ischemic attacks, scientific method, and new realities. Stroke 1991;22:99–104.

12 Baker RN, Broward JA, Fang HC, et al: Anticoagulant therapy of cerebral infarction: report of a national cooperative study. Res Publ Assoc Res Nerv Ment Dis 1966;41:287–302.

13 Acheson J, Hutchinson EC: Observations on the natural history of transient cerebral ischaemia. Lancet 1964;2:871–874.

14 Marshall J: The natural history of transient ischaemic cerebrovascular attacks. Q J Med 1964;33: 309–324.

15 Harrison MJ, Marshall J, Thomas DJ: Relevance of duration of transient ischaemic attacks in carotid territory. BMJ 1978;1:1578–1579.

16 Pessin MS, Duncan GW, Mohr JP, Poskanzer DC: Clinical and angiographic features of carotid transient ischemic attacks. N Engl J Med 1977;296:358–362.

17 Ad Hoc Committee on Cerebrovascular Disease: A classification and outline of cerebrovascular diseases. II. Stroke 1975;6:564–616.

18 National Institute of Neurological Disorders and Stroke rt-PA Stroke Study Group. Tissue plasminogen activator for acute ischemic stroke. N Engl J Med 1995;333:1581–1587.

19 Mohr JP, Biller J, Hilal SK, Yuh WT, Tatemichi TK, Hedges S, Tali E, Nguyen H, Mun I, Adams HP Jr, et al: Magnetic resonance versus computed tomographic imaging in acute stroke. Stroke 1995;26:807–812.

20 Marler JR, Tilley BC, Lu M, et al: Early stroke treatment associated with better outcome: the NINDS rt-PA stroke study. Neurology 2000;55: 1649–1655.

21 Restrepo L, Jacobs MA, Barker PB, Wityk RJ: Assessment of transient ischemic attack with diffusion- and perfusion-weighted imaging. AJNR Am J Neuroradiol 2004;25:1645–1652.

22 Rovira A, Rovira-Gols A, Pedraza S, Grivé E, Molina C, Alvarez-Sabín J: Diffusion-weighted MR imaging in the acute phase of transient ischemic attacks. AJNR Am J Neuroradiol 2002;23:77–83.

23 Mohr JP, Thompson JL, Lazar RM, Levin B, Sacco RL, Furie KL, Kistler JP, Albers GW, Pettigrew LC, Adams HP Jr, Jackson CM, Pullicino P: A comparison of warfarin and aspirin for the prevention of recurrent ischemic stroke. N Engl J Med 2001;345: 1444–1451.

24 Albers GW, Caplan LR, Easton JD, et al: Transient ischemic attack – proposal for a new definition. N Engl J Med 2002;347:1713–1716.

25 Rothwell PM, Giles MF, Flossmann E, et al: A simple score (ABCD) to identify individuals at high early risk of stroke after a transient ischaemic attack. Lancet 2005;366:29–36.

26 Rothwell PM, Buchan A, Johnston SC: Recent advances in the management of transient ischaemic attacks and minor ischaemic stroke. Lancet Neurol 2006;5:323–331.

27 Johnston SC, Rothwell PM, Nguyen-Huynh MN, et al: Validation and refinement of scores to predict very early stroke risk after transient ischaemic attack. Lancet 2007;369:283–292.

28 Luengo-Fernandez R, Gray AM, Rothwell PM: Effect of urgent treatment for transient ischaemic attack and minor stroke on disability and hospital costs (EXPRESS study): a prospective population-based sequential comparison. Lancet Neurol 2009;8:235–243.

29 Rothwell PM, Giles MF, Flossmann E, et al: A simple score (ABCD) to identify individuals at high early risk of stroke after transient ischaemic attack. Lancet 2005;366:29–36.

30 Engelter S, Amort M, Jax F, et al: Optimizing the risk estimation after a transient ischemic attack – The ABCDE+ score. Eur J Neurol 2012;19:55–61.
31 Amort M, Fluri F, Weisskopf F, Gensicke H, Bonati LH, Lyrer PA, Engelter ST: Etiological classifications of transient ischemic attacks: subtype classification by TOAST, CCS and ASCO – a pilot study. Cerebrovasc Dis 2012;33:508–516.
32 Gulli G, Marquardt L, Rothwell PM, Markus HS: Stroke risk after posterior circulation stroke/transient ischemic attack and its relationship to site of vertebrobasilar stenosis: pooled data analysis from prospective studies. Stroke 2013;44:598–604.
33 Lavallee PC, Meseguer E, Abboud H, et al: A transient ischaemic attack clinic with round-the-clock access (SOSTIA): feasibility and effects. Lancet Neurol 2007;6:953–960.
34 Fisher CM: Transient ischemic attacks. N Engl J Med 2002;347:1642–1643.

Prof. Jay P. Mohr
Neurological Institute, Columbia University College of Physicians and Surgeons
710 W. 168th Street
New York, NY 10029 (USA)
E-Mail jpm10@columbia.edu

Uchiyama S, Amarenco P, Minematsu K, Wong KSL (eds): TIA as Acute Cerebrovascular Syndrome.
Front Neurol Neurosci. Basel, Karger, 2014, vol 33, pp 11–18 (DOI: 10.1159/000351888)

The Concept of Acute Cerebrovascular Syndrome

Shinichiro Uchiyama

Department of Neurology, Tokyo Women's Medical University School of Medicine, Tokyo, Japan

Abstract

Early after the onset of transient ischemic attack (TIA), patients are at very high risk of stroke. There is no meaning to differentiate TIA in acute settings from acute ischemic stroke (AIS) only by the duration of symptoms. Acute TIA and AIS are on the same spectrum of acute ischemic syndrome in the central nervous system. We proposed a new concept termed acute cerebrovascular syndrome (ACVS), which includes TIA in acute settings and AIS. The concept of ACVS is comparable to acute coronary syndrome (ACS), which includes unstable angina and acute myocardial infarction. When a focal symptomatic reversible ischemia occurs in the brain, it is called TIA, and when a focal symptomatic irreversible ischemia occurs in the brain, it is called AIS. Patients with ACS share a single pathophysiological mechanism, that is rupture of unstable plaque followed by formation of platelet-rich thrombi to plug up coronary arteries. Unlike ACS, the mechanism of ACVS is complicated, which is not only large artery atherosclerosis similar to ACS but also cardioembolism or small vessel occlusion. In addition, there are no measurable biomarkers for ACVS, while there are practical biomarkers for ACS. Nevertheless, the concept of ACVS is practical to emphasize the importance of immediate evaluation and starting treatment to prevent subsequent stroke in acute settings of TIA. Therefore, TIA in acute settings as well as AIS should be recognized as ACVS, which is a medical emergency.

Importance and Definition of Transient Ischemic Attack

Transient ischemic attack (TIA) is well known to be a prodromal syndrome of ischemic stroke. In reality, 15–30% of patients with ischemic stroke have a history of TIA [1]. Rothwell and Warlow [2] have analyzed 4 studies (Oxford Vascular Study, Oxfordshire Community Stroke Project, UK TIA Aspirin Trial, and European Carotid Surgery Trial), and reported 23% of patients with ischemic stroke had a history of TIA. TIA is, however, easily neglected or underestimated by patients or their families because the symptoms naturally disappear without any treatment. According to a survey in the general population by the Japan Stroke Association, recognition of TIA as a risk

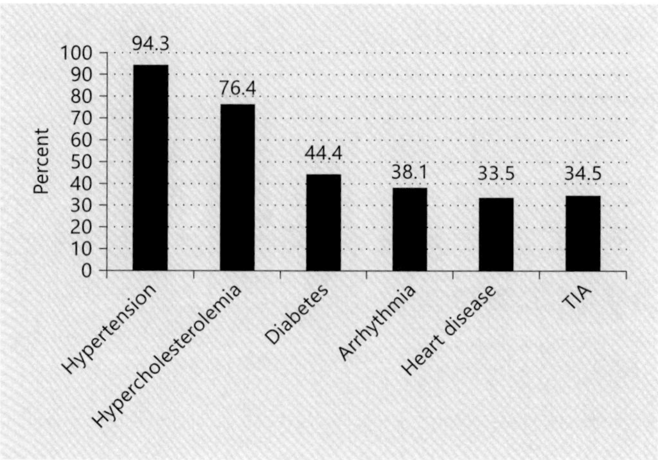

Fig. 1. Recognition of risk factors for stroke in the general population in a survey of the Japan Stroke Association.

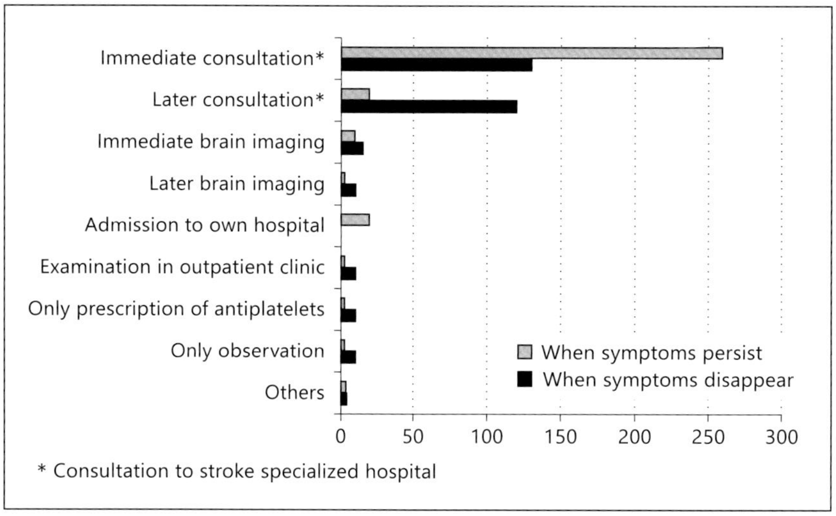

Fig. 2. Survey of general practitioners by the TIA Study Group (Cardiovascular Research of the Japanese Ministry of Health, Labour and Welfare).

factor for stroke was only 34.5%, which was much lower than that of hypertension (94.3%) or hypercholesterolemia (76.4%; fig. 1) [3]. Even by general physicians, TIA is non-prioritized since it is regarded as minor stroke. The TIA Study Group (principal investigator: Kazuo Minematsu) supported by the grant in aid for the Cardiovascular Research from the Japanese Ministry of Health, Labour and Welfare has conducted a survey on the recognition of TIA in general practitioners, and reported that only 42.9% of them answered to immediately consult with stroke-specialized hospitals for patients suspected of TIA in whom the symptoms had disappeared on examination (fig. 2) [4].

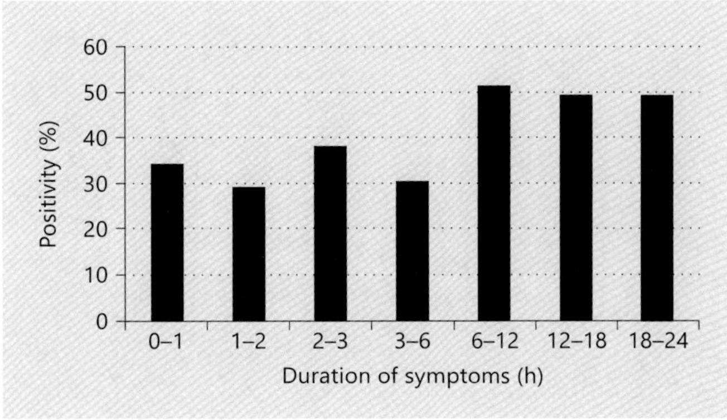

Fig. 3. Duration of neurological symptoms and positivity of DWI. Quoted and modified from Shah et al. [9].

However, TIA patients early after the onset are at very high risk of stroke. According to a population-based study of early risk of stroke after TIA or minor stroke by the Oxford Vascular Study, the estimated risks of recurrent stroke at 7 days, 1 month, and 3 months after a TIA were 8.0, 11.5, and 17.3%, respectively [5]. In addition, it has been reported that in patients who experienced stroke within 2 weeks after the onset of TIA, approximately 30% of stroke cases occurred within 24 h [2]. Therefore, TIA should be recognized to be an emergency requiring immediate evaluation and starting treatment.

There is no global consensus on the definition of TIA. In the classical criteria, TIA is defined as focal neurologic brain or retinal ischemic symptoms which disappear within 24 h [6]. However, the TIA Working Group in the United States defined TIA as brain or retinal ischemic symptoms within 1 h of the duration without responsible ischemic lesions [7]. Afterwards, the American Heart Association/American Stroke Association redefined TIA as transient focal ischemic symptoms in the brain, retina, or spinal cord without evidence of ischemic lesion regardless of the duration of symptoms [8].

New Concept of Acute Cerebral Ischemia

Distribution of the duration of TIA with positive MRI diffusion-weighted image (DWI) is continuous without any specific cutoff point (fig. 3) [9]. A pooled analysis of 808 patients from 10 centers demonstrated that DWI-positive lesions were present in 33%, and these DWI lesions frequently evolve into chronic ischemic lesions on follow-up T2 or fluid-attenuated inversion recovery images [9]. Thus, it is not possible to differentiate TIA from ischemic stroke by symptom duration. Finally, TIA and acute ischemic stroke (AIS) are on the same spectrum of acute ischemic syndrome in the central nervous system.

In the TIAregistry.org (www.tiaregistry.org), which is an international, multicenter cooperative, investigator-driven, web-based observational study, the members in the first

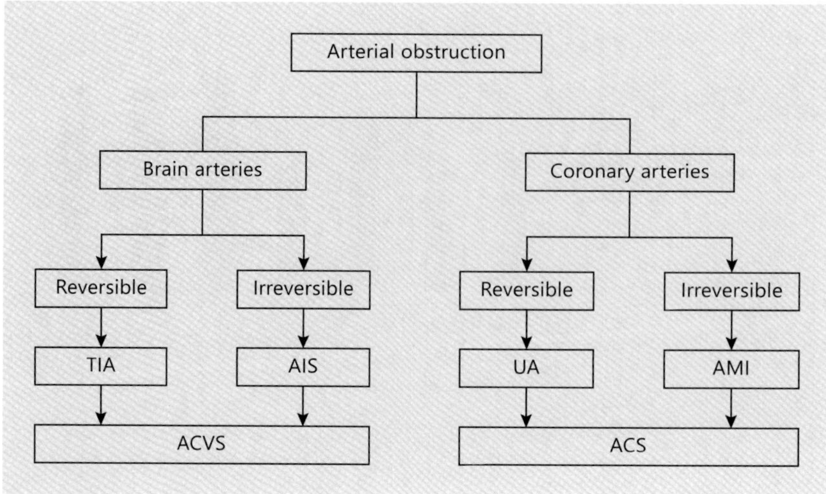

Fig. 4. Concepts of ACVS and ACS.

steering committee meeting (2008 in Paris) proposed a new concept termed acute cerebrovascular syndrome (ACVS), which includes TIA in acute settings and AIS. The concept of ACVS is comparable to acute coronary syndrome (ACS; fig. 4). When a focal symptomatic reversible ischemia occurs in the brain, it is called TIA, and when a focal symptomatic irreversible ischemia occurs in the brain, it is called AIS. On the other hand, when a focal symptomatic reversible ischemia occurs in the heart, it is called unstable angina (UA), and when a focal symptomatic irreversible ischemia occurs in the heart, it is called acute myocardial infarction (AMI). Finally, UA and AMI are categorized into ACS; they share a single pathophysiological mechanism, that is rupture of unstable plaque followed by formation of platelet-rich thrombi to plug up coronary arteries [10, 11].

Unlike ACS, the mechanism of ACVS is complicated, which is not only large artery atherosclerosis similar to ACS but also cardioembolism or small vessel occlusion. In addition, there are no measurable biomarkers for ACVS, while there are practical biomarkers such as troponin T or I as well as electrocardiography for ACS. Nevertheless, the concept of ACVS is practical to emphasize the importance of immediate evaluation and starting treatment to prevent subsequent stroke in acute setting of TIA [12]. Therefore, TIA in acute setting as well as AIS should be recognized as ACVS, which is a medical emergency.

Transient Ischemic Attack as Acute Cerebrovascular Syndrome

There would be no meaning to differentiate TIA from AIS only by the duration of symptoms or MRI positivity. Distribution of the duration is continuous, as shown in figure 5, and MRI positivity is influenced by the timing of imaging. A high-intensity

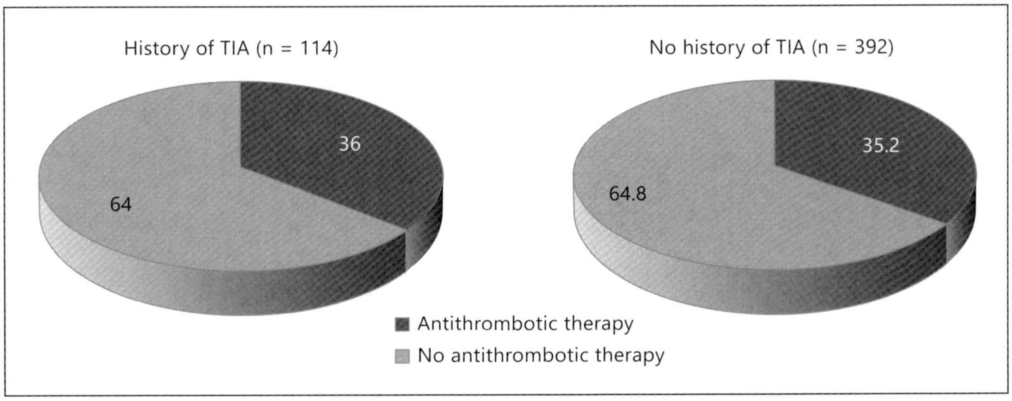

Fig. 5. Prior use of antithrombotics in AIS patients with or without history of TIA. Quoted and modified from Hoshino et al. [17].

lesion may disappear or may newly appear in the follow-up examination. For example, it has been reported that DWI positivity was more frequent in patients who underwent MRI within 24 h of symptom resolution than those imaged after 24 h (37.1 vs. 29.8%; odds ratio, 1.39; 95% confidence interval 1.00–1.93) [9]. On the other hand, Morita et al. [13] have reported that 10 out of 31 (32.3%) patients who did not show positive findings on initial DWI examination showed DWI lesions on the second DWI examination at least 24 h after TIA. Therefore, MRI positivity should be used for a high risk marker of subsequent stroke but not for differentiation of TIA from AIS.

Perfusion studies using MRI or CT may be helpful for detecting a focal ischemic lesion. Two studies have systematically assessed perfusion-weighted MRI (PWI) in the evaluation of TIA patients. In both of these studies, perfusion abnormalities were found in approximately one third of patients, and the frequency of isolated PWI abnormalities without DWI lesions ranged from 3 to 13% [14, 15]. However, it is very difficult to predict whether the focal ischemic lesion is reversible or irreversible, and is consistent or not with the symptoms. Ay et al. [16] reported multiple DWI-positive lesions in 17 of 36 patients with TIA. There does not appear to be a prediction for cortical or subcortical regions or particular vascular territories.

ACVS is a clinical concept but not a pathological diagnosis. The concept of ACVS is important for the recognition of TIA in the acute setting to be a medical emergency as well as AIS. Acute TIA is an unstable cerebral ischemic condition, which is a prodromal symptom before an irreversible thromboembolic event in the brain.

Seven to 40% (15% in average) of stroke patients have a history of TIA [8]. In our retrospective study of 506 consecutive patients with AIS who were admitted to our hospital, 114 (22.5%) patients had a history of stroke [17]. The percentage varies depending on stroke subtypes [8]. In our hospital-based study, it was largest in patients with large artery atherosclerosis (43.9%) and lowest in those with small vessel occlu-

Table 1. Characteristics of patients with TIA who require hospitalization

High clinical risk scores such as ABCD^2 score
Positivity of MRI DWI
Intracranial or extracranial arterial stenosis
Multiple episodes of TIA including crescendo TIA
Non-valvular and valvular atrial fibrillation
Hypercoagulability such as antiphospholipid syndrome

Table 2. Radiological and physiological examinations for initial evaluation of patients with TIA in acute setting

Brain MRI including DWI
Intracranial and extracranial magnetic resonance angiography or computer tomographic angiography
Carotid and vertebral ultrasonography
Electrocardiography with continuous monitoring
Transthoracic and/or transesophageal echocardiography
Transcranial Doppler ultrasound

sion (16.7%) [17]. According to our results, management for stroke prevention was extremely inadequate in the AIS patients with prior history of TIA. This is because antithrombotics had been administered only in approximately one third of AIS patients not only without history of TIA but also with history of TIA, and there was no difference between patients with and without prior TIA (36.6 vs. 35.2%, $p = 0.881$; fig. 5) [17]. The results suggest that TIA is underestimated or overlooked, and even when it was recognized by physicians, they may not recognize the need to give antithrombotics for stroke prevention.

TIA patients in acute settings are at very high risk of subsequent stroke, especially among those with high clinical risk scores such as ABCD^2 score, positivity of diffusion-weighted image, intracranial or extracranial arterial stenosis, multiple episodes of TIA, and hypercoagulability (table 1) [12, 18–20]. The TIA patients with these high risk factors for subsequent stroke should be admitted, and immediate brain and vascular imaging are required as well as blood testing and cardiac evaluation in order to detect vascular and cardiac risk factors (table 2).

After immediate examinations, antithrombotic therapy as well as risk factor management with antihypertensives, statins, and glucose-lowering drugs should be started (table 3) [21]. As to antithrombotic therapy, dual antiplatelet therapy (DAPT) may be effective to prevent early stroke recurrence in patients with non-cardioembolic TIA for aggressive inhibition of platelet activation [22], and novel oral anticoagulants for rapid inhibition of coagulation activation may be useful for preventing early stroke recurrence in patients with cardioembolic TIA due to atrial fibrillation (ta-

Table 3. Initial management in patients with TIA

Management of risk factors
Single or dual antihypertensives
Lipid lowering with statins
Blood glucose-lowering drugs
Antithrombotic therapy
DAPT or single antiplatelet therapy
Novel oral anticoagulants or warfarin
Surgical or intravascular intervention for TIA patients resistant to medical therapy
Carotid endarterectomy
Carotid or vertebral artery stenting
Intracranial bypass surgery

ble 3) [23]. In patients with severe arterial stenosis and resistant to medical treatment, surgical or intravascular intervention with carotid endarterectomy, bypass surgery or carotid artery stenting as an emergency procedure may be necessitated (table 3) [24, 25].

A TIA clinic might be very useful for immediate evaluation and management of acute TIA patients, as it accepts TIA patients 24 h a day, 365 days a year [26]. In reality, according to the results of the EXPRESS study, the TIA clinic was very effective in reducing the risk of stroke during 90 days after TIA [21]. The EXPRESS study showed that this effect was brought about by early starting of DAPT, statin use, and single or dual antihypertensive treatment [21].

In the field of cardiology, ACS terminology including UA and AMI was used for the campaign to save lives from cardiac death, which was very successful in reducing the death rate [27, 28]. In the field of neurology, ACVS terminology is expected to be helpful for reducing the risk of stroke, which is the leading cause of death or disability worldwide [29].

References

1 Hankey GJ, Wardlow CP: Treatment and secondary prevention of stroke: evidence, costs, and effects on individuals and populations. Lancet 1999;354:1457–1463.

2 Rothwell PM, Warlow CP: Timing of TIAs preceding stroke: time window for prevention is very short. Neurology 2005;64:817–820.

3 Miyamatsu N: Epidemiological study on knowledge of stroke and awareness activity by campaign in general people (in Japanese). Report by grant in aid from the Japanese Cardiovascular Research Foundation, 2006, pp 62–67.

4 Suzuki R: Partnership between general physicians and stroke specialized hospitals (in Japanese); in Minematsu K, Uehara T (eds): TIA (Transient Ischemic Attack): Practice of Acute Medical Management. Tokyo, Shindan to Chiryo, 2013, pp 112–117.

5 Coull AJ, Lovett JK, Rothwell PM: Population-based study of early risk of stroke after transient ischaemic attack or minor stroke: implications for public education and organization of services. BMJ 2004;328:326.

6 Special report from the National Institute of Neurological Disorders and Stroke: Classification of cerebrovascular diseases III. Stroke 1990;21:637–676.

7 Albers GW, Caplan LR, Easton JD, et al: Transient ischemic attack: proposal for a new definition. N Engl J Med 2002;347:1713–1716.
8 Easton JD, Saver JL, Albers GW, et al: Definition and evaluation of transient ischemic attack: a scientific statement for healthcare professionals from the American Heart Association/American Stroke Association Stroke Council; Council on Cardiovascular Surgery and Anesthesia; Council on Cardiovascular Radiology and Intervention; Council on Cardiovascular Nursing, and the Interdisciplinary Council on Peripheral Vascular Disease. The American Academy of Neurology affirms the value of this statement as an educational tool for neurologists. Stroke 2009;40:2276–2293.
9 Shah SH, Saver JL, Kidwell CS, et al: A multicenter pooled, patient-level data analysis of diffusion-weighted MRI in TIA patients. Stroke 2007;38:463.
10 Fuster V, Badimon L, Badimon JJ, et al: The pathogenesis of coronary artery disease and the acute coronary syndrome. 1. N Engl J Med 1992;326:242–250.
11 Fuster V, Badimon L, Badimon JJ, et al: The pathogenesis of coronary artery disease and the acute coronary syndrome. 2. N Engl J Med 1992;326:310–318.
12 Johnston SC, Nquyen-Huynh MN, Schwarz ME, et al: National Stroke Association guidelines for the management of transient ischemic attacks. Ann Neurol 2006;60:301–313.
13 Morita N, Harada M, Satomi J, et al: Frequency of emerging positive diffusion-weighted imaging in early repeat examinations at least 24 h transient ischemic attacks. Neuroradiology 2013;55:399–403.
14 Restrepo L, Jacobs MA, Barker PB, et al: Assessment of transient ischemic attack with diffusion- and perfusion-weighted imaging. AJNR Am J Neuroradiol 2004;25:1645–1652.
15 Krol AI, Coutts SB, Simon JE, et al, for the VSION Study Group: Perfusion MRI abnormalities in speech or motor transient ischemic attack patients. Stroke 2005;36:2487–2489.
16 Ay H, Koroshetz WJ, Benner T, et al: Transient ischemic attack with infarction: a unique syndrome? Ann Neurol 2005;57:679–686.
17 Hoshino T, Mizuno S, Shimizu S, Uchiyama S: Clinical features and functional outcome of stroke after transient ischemic attack. J Stroke Cerebrovasc Dis 2013;22:260–266.
18 Johnston SC, Rothwell PM, Nguyen-Huynh MN, et al: Validation and refinement of score to predict very early stroke risk after transient ischaemic attack. Lancet 2007;369:283–292.
19 Giles MF, Albers GW, Amarenco P, et al: Addition of brain infarction to the ABCD^2 score (ABCD^{2}I): a collaborative analysis of unpublished data on 4,574 patients. Stroke 2010;41:1907–1913.
20 Merwick A, Albers GW, Amarenco P, et al: Addition of brain and carotid imaging to the ABCD^2 score to identify patients at early risk of stroke after transient ischaemic attack: a multicenter observational study. Lancet Neurol 2010;9:1060–1069.
21 Rothwell PM, Matthew FG, Chandratheva A, et al: Effect of urgent treatment of transient ischaemic attack and minor stroke on early recurrent stroke (EXPRES study): a prospective population-based sequential comparison. Lancet 2007;370:1432–1442.
22 Wang Y, Johnston SC: Clopidogrel and aspirin versus aspirin alone for acute TIA and minor stroke. N Engl J Med 2013;369:11–19.
23 Uchiyama S, Ibayashi S, Matsumoto M, et al: Dabigatran and factor Xa inhibitors for stroke prevention in patients with nonvalvular atrial fibrillation. J Stroke Cerebrovasc Dis 2012;21:165–173.
24 Furie KL, Kasner SE, Adams RJ, et al: Guidelines for the prevention of stroke in patients with stroke or transient ischemic attack. A guideline for healthcare professionals from the American Heart Association/America Stroke Association. Stroke 2011;42:227–276.
25 Brott TG, Halperin JL, Abbara S, et al: 2011 ASA/ACCF/AHA/AANN/AANS/ACR/ASNR/CNS/SAIP/SCAI/SIR/SVM/SVS guideline on the management of patients with extracranial carotid and vertebral artery disease: executive summary. Catheter Cardiovasc Interv 2013;81:E76–E123.
26 Lavallee PC, Meseguer E, Abboud H, et al: A transient ischaemic attack clinic with round-the-clock access (SOS-TIA): feasibility and effects. Lancet Neurol 2007;6:953–960.
27 Steg PG, Bonnefoy E, Chabaud S, et al: Impact of time to treatment on mortality after prehospital fibrinolysis or primary angioplasty: data from the CAPTIM randomized clinical trial. Circulation 2003;108:2851–2856.
28 O'Conner RE, Brady W, Brooks SC, et al: Part 10: acute coronary syndromes. 2010 American Heart Association Guidelines for cardiopulmonary resuscitation and emergency cardiovascular care. Circulation 2010;122(suppl):S787–S817.
29 Strong K, Mathers C: The global burden of stroke; in Mohr JP, Wolf PA, Grotta JC, et al (eds): Stroke: Pathophysiology, Diagnosis, and Management, ed 5. Philadelphia, Elsevier Saunders, 2011, pp 279–289.

Prof. Shinichiro Uchiyama, MD, PhD
Department of Neurology, Tokyo Women's Medical University School of Medicine
8-1 Kawada-cho, Shinjuku-ku
Tokyo 162-8666 (Japan)
E-Mail suchiyam@nij.twmu.ac.jp

Uchiyama S, Amarenco P, Minematsu K, Wong KSL (eds): TIA as Acute Cerebrovascular Syndrome.
Front Neurol Neurosci. Basel, Karger, 2014, vol 33, pp 19–29 (DOI: 10.1159/000351889)

Transient Ischemic Attack as a Medical Emergency

Yasushi Okada

Department of Cerebrovascular Medicine and Neurology and Clinical Research Institute, National Hospital Organization Kyushu Medical Center, Fukuoka, Japan

Abstract

Since transient ischemic attack (TIA) is regarded as a medical emergency with high risk for early stroke recurrence, the underlying mechanisms should be immediately clarified to conclude a definitive diagnosis and provide early treatment. Early risk stratification using $ABCD^2$ scores can predict the risk of ischemic stroke occurring after TIA. Carotid ultrasonography (US) can evaluate the degree of stenosis, plaque properties and flow velocity of ICA lesions. High-risk mobile plaques can be classified by carotid US, and aortogenic sources of emboli can be detected by transesophageal echocardiography. Cardiac monitoring and blood findings are thought to play a key role in a diagnosis of cardioembolic TIA. Diffusion-weighted imaging (DWI)-MRI and MR angiography are also indispensable to understand the mechanism of TIA and cerebral circulation. To prevent subsequent stroke arising from TIA, antiplatelet and anticoagulant therapies should be started immediately along with comprehensive management of life-style, hypertension, diabetes mellitus, dyslipidemia and other atherosclerotic diseases. Carotid endarterectomy and endovascular intervention are critical for treating symptomatic patients with significant stenosis of ICA. A novel concept of acute cerebrovascular syndrome (ACVS) has recently been advocated to increase awareness of TIA among citizens, patients and medical professionals. TIA should be recognized as the last opportunity to avoid irreversible ischemic stroke and its sequelae. The clinical relevance of the new concept of ACVS is advocated by early recurrence after TIA, analysis of high-risk TIA, treatment strategies and the optimal management of TIA. Raising TIA awareness should also proceed across many population sectors.

Urgency: Short-Term Risk of Transient Ischemic Attack

Patients with transient ischemic attacks (TIAs) are at high risk of early stroke. Large cohort and population-based studies over the past decade have demonstrated a higher risk of early stroke after TIA than had been suspected. In general, 15–20% of patients have a stroke within 3 months of a TIA [1], with half of those occurring within

48 h [2]. Several recent guidelines recommend that patients with TIA should be thoroughly assessed within 24 h. In a prospective, population-based observation with complete follow-up (Oxford Vascular Study) of 1,247 patients with a first TIA or stroke, 35 had recurrent stroke in the same arterial territory within 24 h. The 6-, 12-, and 24-hour stroke risks after 488 first TIAs are 1.2, 2.1 and 5.1%, respectively, and 42% of all recurrent strokes during the 30 days after a first TIA occur within the first 24 h [3]. The 12- and 24-hour risk area is closely associated with $ABCD^2$ scores. Recurrent strokes within the first 24 h of a TIA highlight the need for emergency assessment. The $ABCD^2$ score is a reliable clinical indicator during the acute phase to assess appropriate triage, emergency management and feasible treatment. However, most patients with TIA do not receive optimal treatment even today; statins are not administered, and blood pressure is not controlled. Many patients are prescribed with aspirin and sent home directly from an emergency room without additional evaluation. Yet risk is particularly high during the first few days after TIA. Studies in northern California (USA) and Oxfordshire (UK) found an approximate 4% risk of stroke within the first 24 h of a TIA, which is about twice the risk of myocardial infarction or death in patients presenting with acute coronary syndrome (about 2% at 24 h). The northern California study followed up 1,707 patients for 3 months after a first visit to an emergency room where they were diagnosed with TIA. The results showed an unexpectedly high (10.5%) overall incidence of stroke during the 3-month period, and half of these developed within 48 h after the onset of TIA [4]. Recurrent ischemic stroke occurred in 8 (5%) of 160 consecutive patients with DWI-negative TIA during hospitalization at Kyushu Medical Center [5]. All of these occurred within 7 days with a median of 2.5 days. Unlike the German Stroke Bank study [6], a lacunar etiology was the most frequent, and modified Rankin Scale outcomes were mostly good at discharge (fig. 1a). The incidence of recurrent stroke closely correlates with $ABCD^2$ score. The prevalence of both atrial fibrillation (AF) and occlusive arterial disease is also significantly higher in patients with, than without recurrent stroke. An atherothrombotic etiology is more likely in the unclassified type (AF and/or middle cerebral artery), since PT-INR in these types remains within the optimal range (fig. 1b). These results are particularly characteristic in Japan, compared with USA-European findings. Even under immediate best medical management, patients with high $ABCD^2$ scores tended to develop recurrent stroke. A combination of AF and occlusive arterial disease might indicate high risk for early recurrence of ischemic stroke in patients with TIA.

Effect of Emergency Care

The EXPRESS (Early use of EXisting PREventive Strategies for Stroke) study [7] in Oxford (UK) was designed to compare the outcomes of treatment before and after switching to emergency care in which each patient is evaluated more actively and urgently at a TIA clinic and treatment with proven methods is started within 24 h when

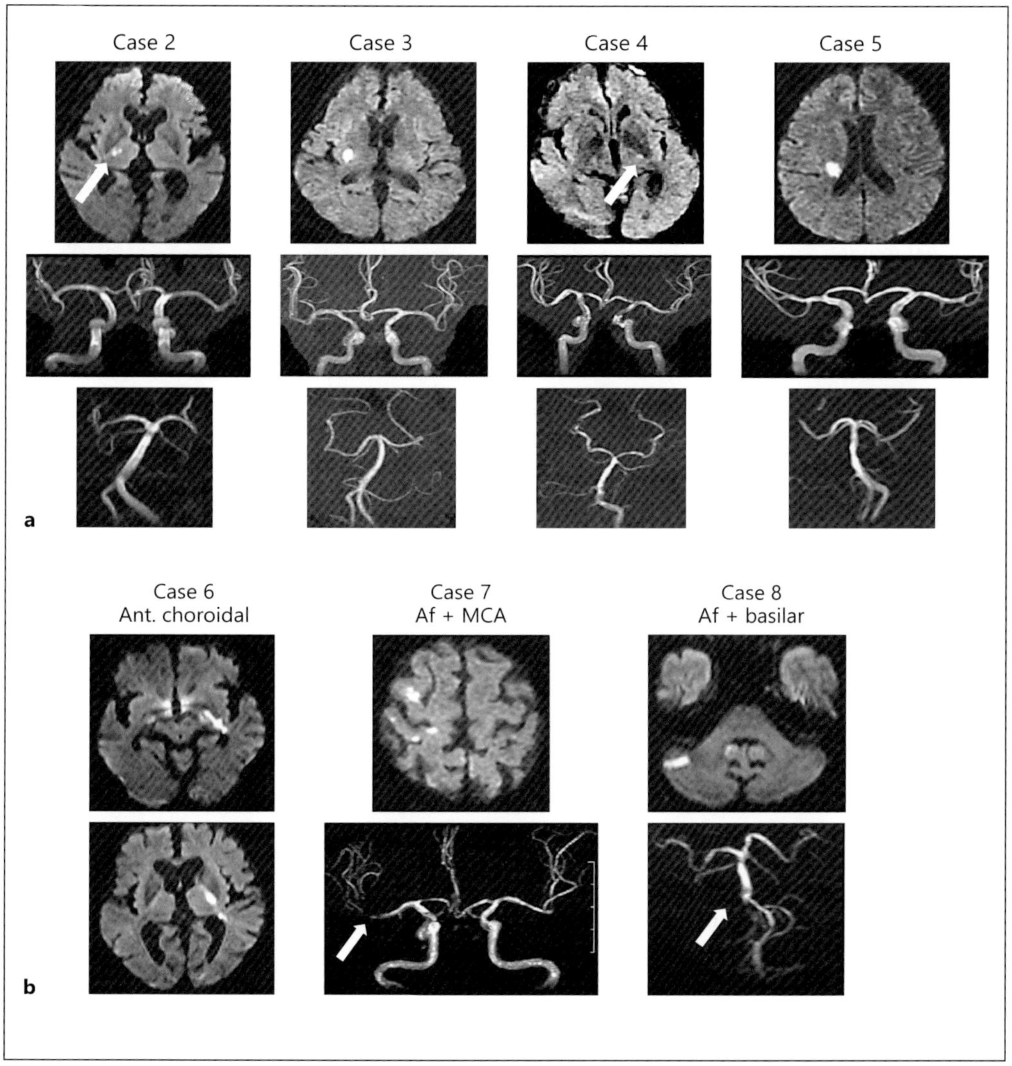

Fig. 1. Recurrent brain infarction in patients with DWI-negative TIA of unclassified and lacunar etiology. Four patients with lacunar TIA (**a**) and 3 with unclassified TIA accompanied by AF and intracranial artery disease (**b**). Modified from Mori et al. [27].

possible. The findings showed that early treatment positively affected socioeconomic outcomes, length of hospital stay and reduced the incidence of ischemic stroke and improved activities of daily living (ADL) at 90 days [7, 8]. Although these were observational studies and the influence from confounding factors could not be ruled out, the stroke risk after onset of TIA or minor ischemic stroke decreased by 80% compared with risk recorded before starting emergency care. Lavallée et al. [9] also evaluated the effects of rapidly assessing patients with TIA at a TIA clinic on clinical decision-making, the length of hospital stay and subsequent stroke rates. Patients were

Fig. 2. Treatment on same spectrum as acute ischemic attack. Awareness of TIA as ACVS that requires emergency examination and treatment, like acute coronary syndrome.

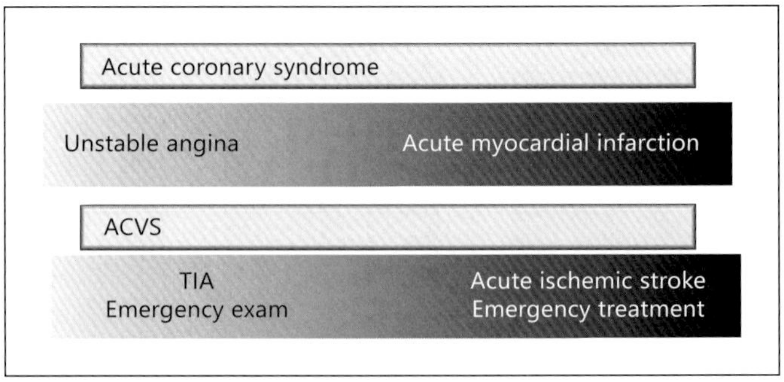

assessed within 4 h of admission by means that included neurological, arterial and cardiac imaging. Among 1,085 patients admitted with suspected TIA, 574 (53%) attended the TIA clinic within 24 h of symptom onset, 701 (65%) had confirmed TIA or minor stroke, and 144 (13%) had possible TIA. Of the patients with confirmed or possible TIA, all started a stroke prevention program, 43 (5%) had urgent carotid revascularization, and 44 (5%) were treated for AF with anticoagulants. After assessment, 808 (74%) of the patients seen were sent home on the same day. The 90-day stroke rate was 1.24% (95% CI: 0.72–2.12), whereas the rate predicted from $ABCD^2$ scores was 5.96%. This 80% stroke reduction was exactly the same as the EXPRESS results, that is, risk predicted based on $ABCD^2$ scores. Use of TIA clinics with 24-hour access and the immediate initiation of preventive treatment might greatly reduce length of hospital stay and risk of stroke compared with predicted risk. Thus, this type of emergency TIA clinic is very effective in preventing stroke. The results of the EXPRESS and SOS-TIA registry referred to the 2009 Japanese Guidelines for the Management of Stroke [10], which state, 'If TIA is suspected, the onset mechanism should be identified as soon as possible, and treatment to prevent subsequent cerebral infarction must be started immediately (Grade A)'. Since the early intensive management of TIA is rather important and awareness of TIA as a medical emergency needs to be heightened, a new concept of acute cerebrovascular syndrome (ACVS) that requires emergency examinations and treatment has been advocated along the lines of acute coronary syndrome [11] (fig. 2).

Acute cardioembolic brain infarction without prior TIA is not rare, and often results in severe and irreversible neurological deficits that are referred to as devastating or knockout brain infarction, implying a bedridden state brought about by one straight punch delivered by a cardiac embolus. About 1.6–20% of patients with cardioembolic stroke reportedly experience recurrent stroke in another vascular territory within 2 weeks [12, 13]. Therefore, if AF is detected in patients with TIA in the acute setting, anticoagulant therapy should be started as soon as possible because prior TIA is a red flag indicating a last chance to avoid severe neurological impairment.

Carotid artery stenosis is responsible for crescendo TIA and stroke. In practice, the North American Symptomatic Carotid Endarterectomy Trial (NASCET) found an

8.9 and 20.1% incidence of ipsilateral stroke during 7 and 90 days, respectively, after TIA onset in patients with carotid artery severe stenosis [14]. Bond et al. [15] reported that the prognosis of patients with TIA accompanied by carotid stenosis differs greatly depending on whether or not treatment is provided within 2 weeks of disease onset. However, the reality is that carotid endarterectomy (CEA) and stenting often proceed several weeks after onset.

Key Points of Risk Stratification at First Visit

What are the early risks of stroke and other vascular outcomes? Northern California studies found that adverse events including admission for cardiovascular events, death, and recurrent TIA occurred in 25.1% of patients studied during 3 months after the onset of a TIA. The $ABCD^2$ score was derived to provide a more standard prediction and it incorporates elements from both prior scores. In combined validation cohorts, the 2-day risk of stroke was 0% for scores of 0 or 1, 1.3% for 2 or 3, 4.1% for 4 or 5, and 8.1% for 6 or 7 in the summation of following factors: age ≥60 years (1), blood pressure ≥140/90 mm Hg on first evaluation, clinical symptoms of focal weakness with spelling (2) or speech impairment without weakness; duration ≥60 min (2) or 10–59 min (1) and diabetes (1). The 2-day period after TIA onset is critical for determining whether a patient should be hospitalized or managed as an outpatient in a non-timely fashion (with some delay) [16]. On the other hand, patients with apparently low-risk TIA-like symptoms should also be evaluated for early risk after an attack. Among 907 patients presenting with dizziness, cerebrovascular conditions were the cause in 37 (4.1%), and most of them were ischemic strokes (n = 24). The $ABCD^2$ score predicted that an ultimate cerebrovascular event might provide useful information about dizziness in patients presenting at emergency department who are at low risk for a cerebrovascular diagnosis [17]. These findings underscore the need for the prompt evaluation and treatment of patients with symptoms of ischemia.

The presence of a new infarct on brain images, which is consistent with the classic definition of TIA but would not lead to stroke, is associated with about a 2- to 15-fold increase in the subsequent short-term risk of stroke. Evidence of vessel occlusion on acute brain MRA also has been associated with a 4-fold increased short-term risk of stroke [18, 19]. A total of 159 patients were enrolled in a study of silent new DWI lesions within the first week after a stroke [20]. Clinical stroke recurrence was detected in 2.5% of these patients. A new cerebral lesion was detected in 5.7% of patients between a first and a second imaging assessment (first interval) and in 23.3% between a second and a third imaging assessment (second interval). Multivariable analysis has independently associated new lesions with ipsilateral carotid stenosis, recanalization and a multiple lesion pattern. New lesions on DWI arise more often than routine neurological examination suggests. Stroke risk immediately after TIA defined by time-based criteria is high, and prognostic scores ($ABCD^2$ and $ABCD^3$-I) have been devel-

Table 1. Treatment policy for TIA

Immediate hospitalization; treated as for acute brain infarct
ABCD^2 score ≥3 points
Initial attack within 3 days
Frequent or multiple TIA
Cardioembolic TIA
Advanced carotid stenosis
Sustained symptoms
Cerebral cortical symptoms
Outpatient examinations; anti-platelet therapy
Single attack: hospital visit 1–2 weeks later
Elective hospitalization for detailed examination
Cardiogenic or main artery lesion or high risk for TIA found on outpatient basis

oped to assist management. Among patients with lesions on DWI, recurrent stroke rates at 7 days after tissue-negative and -positive events were 7.1 and 0.4%, respectively. The ABCD^2 score had a predictive value in tissue-positive and -negative events [20]. These findings support the concept of a tissue-based definition of TIA and stroke, at least on prognostic grounds.

Hospitalization: Transient Ischemic Attack Management Policy

Hospitalization rates after TIA vary widely among practitioners, hospitals, and regions. A study from the National Hospital Ambulatory Medical Care Survey found that 54% of patients with TIA were admitted to a hospital, with rates varying from 68% in the northwest United States of America to 41% in the west. Over 70% of patients with TIA in the acute setting are admitted to our hospital, like other specialized stroke hospitals in Japan. An ABCD^2 score of >3 points is currently applied to make initial decisions regarding hospital admission. A history of frequent TIAs, cardioembolic TIA, carotid stenosis of >50% on the ischemic side, typical symptoms lasting >60 min, cerebral cortical symptoms such as aphasia and hemianopsia are thought to indicate high-risk TIA that warrants admission. On the other hand, patients who present several days after TIA onset are examined and treated on an outpatient basis using antiplatelets unless a cardiogenic source or main artery lesion is detected (table 1). The recommended initial examination for TIA after taking a medical history comprises physical and neurological examinations, ECG, blood tests including CBC, biochemistry, prothrombin time/activated partial tromboplastin time, lipid and blood sugars, and MRI to detect new ischemic lesions and vascular stenosis. DWI-MRI is essential in Japan. Noninvasive examinations such as carotid ultrasound, MRA and

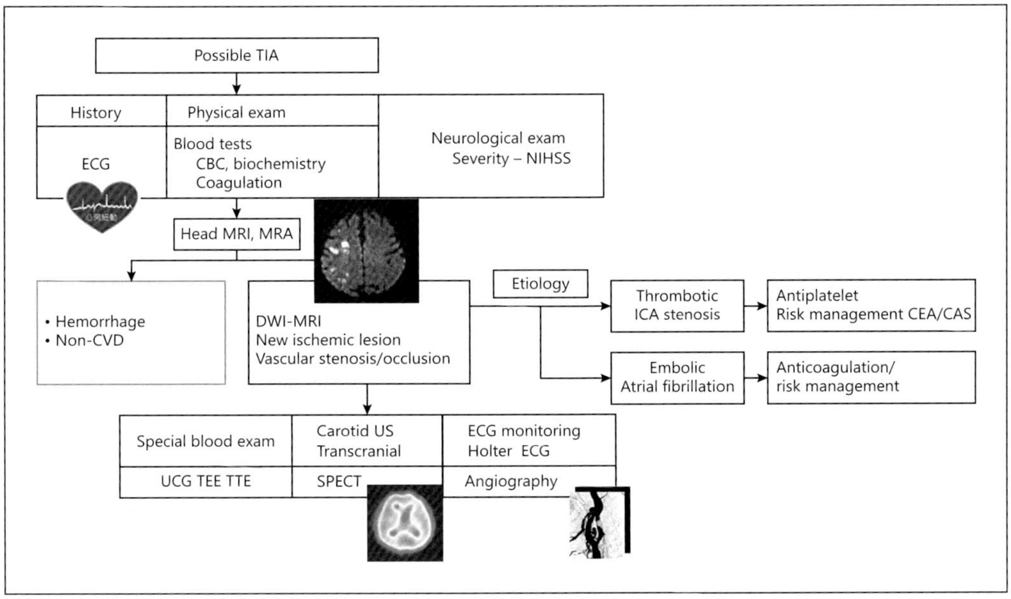

Fig. 3. Initial immediate screening for ACVS.

CT angiography are initially recommended to detect vascular stenosis. Such examinations should be completed by the end of the first outpatient or admission day. ECG monitoring, Holter ECG and specific blood tests such as brain natriuretic peptide and D-dimer are also simultaneously recommended to confirm cardioembolic etiology in specialized clinics. To detect paroxysmal AF (PAF), repeated, long monitoring ECG is essential. If necessary, cerebral angiography and single photon emission tomography are used to measure cerebral blood flow during hospitalization (fig. 3).

Plaque properties must be evaluated before vascular reconstruction to treat symptomatic severe carotid stenosis. The degree of stenosis and flow velocity is examined using carotid ultrasonography (US), and then plaque properties are determined using US and MRI. Unstable plaque at the origin of the ICA can be detected on US, MPRAGE or by the black blood method using MRI. Low echoic mobile plaque, a thin fibrous cap, and ulcer formation determined by carotid US indicate high risk for subsequent ischemic attacks. Mobile plaques have been defined (fig. 4) as the jellyfish type, on which a thin fibrous cap fluctuates, the streaming band type, in which swaying fibers are attached to the plaque, the mobile thrombus type, in which a mobile mass is attached to the plaque surface, and the fluctuating ulcer type, which contains mobile substances and an ulcer. The rate of early recurrence is significantly higher in patients with mobile than non-mobile plaques [22]. Intracranial collateral circulation is evaluated by MRA and calcified lesions are determined by CT angiography. Cardiac examinations to detect significant coronary disease such as SPECT are also necessary before any surgery. A final diagnosis is confirmed by DSA. In summary, severe ICA

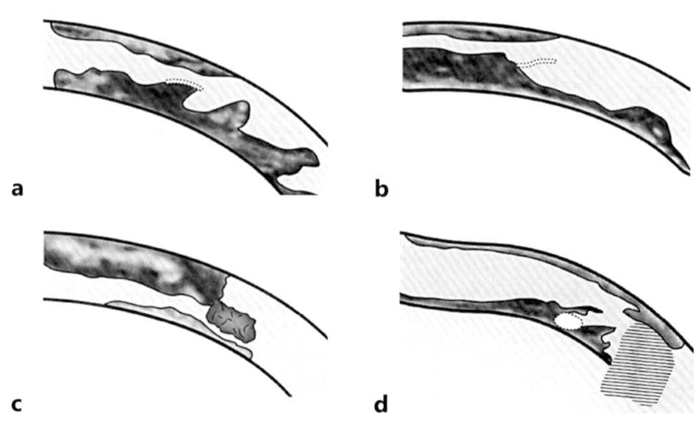

Fig. 4. Morphological classification of mobile plaques. Jellyfish (**a**), streaming band (**b**), mobile thrombus (**c**) and fluctuating ulcer (**d**) types. Rate of mobile plaque: 12.8% in 94 acute-stroke patients. From Ogata et al. [22].

stenosis with unstable mobile plaques are closely associated with early stroke recurrence. Immediate secondary prevention, optimal perioperative medical treatment, and standardized operative techniques have enabled neurologically stable patients with TIAs to undergo CEA/carotid artery stenting as an acceptable risk of stroke. Further study of the relationships between procedural risk and the timing of surgery is required.

Close observation during hospitalization has the potential to allow more rapid and frequent administration of tissue plasminogen activator should a stroke occur. Hospitalization might also confer other benefits derived from cardiac monitoring and rapid diagnostic evaluation. A recent study identified AF during the early phase of cryptogenic ischemic stroke, indicating that such patients might have undetected PAF. The Stroke and Monitoring for PAF in Real Time (SMART) registry was established to determine the yield of 30-day outpatient PAF monitoring in patients with cryptogenic ischemic stroke [23]. An intent-to-monitor analysis detected PAF in 29 of 239 patients (12.1%; 95% CI: 8.6–16.9%). After a retrospective chart review, a new diagnosis of PAF was confirmed in 26 of 236 patients (11.0%; 95% CI: 7.6–15.7). Most of the detected PAF events were asymptomatic, and only 6 of 98 recorded PAF events (6.1%) were patient triggered or associated with symptoms. About 1 in 9 patients with cryptogenic ischemic stroke have new PAF within 30 days. Routine monitoring in this population should be recommended. A report from the National Cardiovascular Center indicated that patients with TIA accompanied by AF are slightly older, smoke less frequently, have less frequent episodes of TIA (one episode on average) and an obviously higher incidence of aphasia than TIA patients without AF [24]. No randomized trials have yet evaluated the benefit of hospitalization or the utility of the $ABCD^2$ score in assisting with triage decisions. In-hospital mortality was higher for patients with cardioembolic stroke (10.0% in our series) than with any other subtypes of cerebral infarction. Secondary prevention with anticoagulants should be started immediately in patients at high risk for recurrent cardioembolic stroke in which contraindications such as poor compliance or gastrointestinal bleeding are absent. Dabigatran and rivaroxaban are useful to immediately prevent recurrent embolic attacks in TIA patients with AF and are recommended for patient with AF. These agents are not only similar to warfarin in their ability to prevent stroke or systemic embolism, but they can also lower the incidence of intracranial hemorrhage more effectively.

Importance of Awareness of Transient Ischemic Attack

No consensus about primary care has been reached in Japan regarding how to manage patients with TIA. Patients diagnosed with TIA are simply prescribed with aspirin and sent home directly from the emergency room. Medical staff will often regard TIA as a trivial transient neurological event and a different clinical entity from acute ischemic stroke. Moreover, almost all citizens are unaware of the risk of TIA and its clinical relevance. Awareness of TIA as an ACVS that requires early management like acute coronary syndrome must be disseminated. Citizens should understand the high risk of subsequent stroke during the first several hours after TIA onset and that the risk cannot be controlled unless treatment is started before a stroke occurs. Thus, citizens should be educated about treating TIA as soon as possible and to take instant action from all viewpoints [25], including immediate presentation at a TIA clinic. Educational campaigns are needed to teach citizens about the higher prevalence of comorbid diseases, such as hypertension (65 vs. 39%), diabetes mellitus (26 vs. 15%), and dyslipidemia (29 vs. 27%) in patients with TIA and carotid stenosis, than in those without. Most studies have found that less than half of stroke/TIA events result in a 911 call. One study found that 40% of 2,975 patients with stroke/TIA who met inclusion criteria used emergency medical services [26]. After adjustment, the symptoms that increased the odds of a 911 call were weakness, confusion/decreased level of consciousness, speech/language, and dizziness/coordination/vertigo. Numbness was less likely to result in a 911 call as were visual changes. The public appears to respond differently based on the type of stroke symptom, regardless of overall severity. Public awareness messages regarding stroke warning signs should be designed with this in mind. In addition, leaflets about TIA with toll-free telephone numbers for TIA clinics have been sent to family doctors, cardiologists, neurologists and ophthalmologists in various areas and their administrative regions [9]. The effect of increasing TIA awareness through media campaigns in the city of Fukuoka on changes in public behavior has been examined by the Kyushu Medical Center group using an on-line survey. The respondents were 618 individuals with no history of stroke living in Fukuoka prefecture. Pre- and post-surveys were conducted in March and June 2011, respectively. Awareness of TIA as a medical emergency and a risk factor in subsequent stroke was spread in newspapers, magazines, banners and transit advertising as well as at public events, and on the radio and TV over a 2-month period. Among 608 respondents, 72 (11.7%) had seen and 131 (21.2%) might have seen the advertisements. Newspaper,

TV, and hospital posters seemed particularly effective. A comparison of individual attitudes before and after the advertising campaign showed that those who had seen the ads checked the disease information, consulted with others and attended hospitals or clinics more frequently than those without the exposure to the campaign. A nation-wide educational campaign should focus on raising awareness of high-risk TIA using $ABCD^2$ scores and reducing stroke recurrence.

References

1 Wu CM, McLaughlin K, Lorenzetti DL, Hill MD, Manns BJ, Ghali WA: Early risk of stroke after transient ischemic attack: a systematic review and meta-analysis. Arch Intern Med 2007;167:2417–2422.

2 Lisabeth LD, Ireland JK, Risser JM, Brown DL, Smith MA, Garcia NM, et al: Stroke risk after transient ischemic attack in a population-based setting. Stroke 2004;35:1842–1846.

3 Chandratheva A, Mehta Z, Geraghty OC, Marquardt L, Rothwell PM: Population-based study of risk and predictors of stroke in the first few hours after a TIA. Neurology 2009;72:1941–1947.

4 Johnston SC, Gress DR, Browner WS, Sidney S: Short-term prognosis after emergency department diagnosis of TIA. JAMA 2000;284:2901–2906.

5 Mori M, Okada Y, Yoshimura S, Matsushita T, Miyazaki Y, Makihara N, Wakugawa Y, Yasaka M: ABCD2 score to identify individuals on admission at high early risk of stroke after transient ischemic attack. Jpn J Stroke 2011;33:25–30.

6 Weimar C, Kraywinkel K, Rödl J, Hippe A, Harms L, Kloth A, Diener HC; German Stroke Data Bank Collaborators: Etiology, duration, and prognosis of transient ischemic attacks: an analysis from the German Stroke Data Bank. Arch Neurol 2002;59:1584–1588.

7 Rothwell PM, Giles MF, Chandratheva A, Marquardt L, Geraghty O, Redgrave JN, et al: Effect of urgent treatment of transient ischaemic attack and minor stroke on early recurrent stroke (EXPRESS study): a prospective population-based sequential comparison. Lancet 2007;370:1432–1442.

8 Luengo-Fernandez R, Gray AM, Rothwell PM: Effect of urgent treatment for transient ischaemic attack and minor stroke on disability and hospital costs (EXPRESS study): a prospective population-based sequential comparison. Lancet Neurol 2009;8:235–243.

9 Lavallée PC, Meseguer E, Abboud H, Cabrejo L, Olivot JM, Simon O, et al: A transient ischaemic attack clinic with round-the-clock access (SOS-TIA): feasibility and effects. Lancet Neurol 2007;6:953–960.

10 Shinohara Y, Yanagihara T, Abe K, Yoshimine T, Fujinaka T, Chuma T, Ochi F, Nagayama M, Ogawa A, Suzuki N, Katayama Y, Kimura A, Minematsu K: II. Cerebral infarction/transient ischemic attack (TIA). J Stroke Cerebrovasc Dis 2011;20(suppl 1):S31–S73.

11 Uchiyama S, Johnston SC, Okada Y: New concepts of treatment for TIA as a medical emergency (round table discussion). Int Rev Thromb 2009;4:5–21.

12 Guedes LC, Ferro JM: A systematic review of immediate anticoagulation for ischemic stroke of presumed cardioembolic origin. Stroke 2008;39:e81–e82.

13 Paciaroni M, Agnelli G, Micheli S, Caso V: Efficacy and safety of anticoagulant treatment in acute cardioembolic stroke: a meta-analysis of randomized controlled trials. Stroke 2007;38:423–430.

14 Eliasziw M, Kennedy J, Hill MD, Buchan AM, Barnett HJM, The North American Symptomatic Carotid Endarterectomy Trial (NASCET) Group: Early risk of stroke after a transient ischemic attack in patients with internal carotid artery disease. CMAJ 2004;170:1105–1109.

15 Bond R, Rerkasem K, Rothwell PM: Systematic review of the risks of carotid endarterectomy in relation to the clinical indication for and timing of surgery. Stroke 2003;34:2290–2301.

16 Johnston SC, Rothwell PM, Nguyen-Huynh MN, Giles MF, Elkins JS, Bernstein AL, et al: Validation and refinement of scores to predict very early stroke risk after transient ischaemic attack. Lancet 2007;369:283–292.

17 Navi BB, Kamel H, Shah MP, Grossman AW, Wong C, Poisson SN, Whetstone WD, Josephson SA, Johnston SC, Kim AS: Application of the ABCD2 score to identify cerebrovascular causes of dizziness in the emergency department. Stroke 2012;43:1484–1489.

18 Purroy F, Montaner J, Rovira A, Delgado P, Quintana M, Alvarez-Sabin J: Higher risk of further vascular events among transient ischemic attack patients with diffusion-weighted imaging acute ischemic lesions. Stroke 2004;35:2313–2319.

19 Calvet D, Touze E, Oppenheim C, Turc G, Meder JF, Mas JL: DWI lesions and TIA etiology improve the prediction of stroke after TIA. Stroke 2009;40:187–192.
20 Nolte CH, Albach FN, Heuschmann PU, Brunecker P, Villringer K, Endres M, Fiebach JB: Silent new DWI lesions within the first week after stroke. Cerebrovasc Dis 2012;33:248–254.
21 Giles MF, Albers GW, Amarenco P, Arsava EM, Asimos AW, Ay H, Calvet D, Coutts SB, Cucchiara BL, Demchuk AM, Johnston SC, Kelly PJ, Kim AS, Labreuche J, Lavallee PC, Mas J-L, Merwick A, Olivot JM, Purroy F, Rosamond WD, Sciolla R, Rothwell PM: Early stroke risk and ABCD2 score performance in tissue- vs time-defined TIA. A multicenter study. Neurology 2011;77:1222–1228.
22 Ogata T, Yasaka M, Wakugawa Y, Kitazono T, Okada Y: Morphological classification of mobile plaques and their association with early recurrence of stroke. Cerebrovasc Dis 2010;30:606–611.
23 Flint AC, Banki NM, Ren X, Rao VA, Go AS: Detection of paroxysmal atrial fibrillation by 30-day event monitoring in cryptogenic ischemic stroke: the Stroke and Monitoring for PAF in Real Time (SMART) Registry. Stroke 2012;43:2788–2790.
24 Inoue T, Kimura K, Minematsu K, Yamaguchi T, Japan Multicenter Stroke Investigators' Collaboration (J-MUSIC: Clinical features of transient ischemic attack associated with atrial fibrillation: analysis of 1084 TIA patients. J Stroke Cerebrovasc Dis 2004;13:155–159.
25 Coull AJ, Lovett JK, Rothwell PM; Oxford Vascular Study: Population based study of early risk of stroke after transient ischaemic attack or minor stroke: implications for public education and organisation of services. BMJ 2004;328:326–328.
26 Kleindorfer D, Lindsell CJ, Moomaw CJ, Alwell K, Woo D, Flaherty ML, Adeoye O, Zakaria T, Broderick JP, Kissela BM: Which stroke symptoms prompt a 911 call? A population-based study. Am J Emerg Med 2010;28:607–612.
27 Mori M, Okada Y, Yoshimura S, Matsushita T, Miyazaki Y, Makihara N, Wakugawa Y, Yasaka M: ABCD2 score to identify individuals on admission at high early risk of stroke after transient ischemic attack. Jpn J Stroke 2011;33:25–30.

Yasushi Okada, MD, PhD
Department of Cerebrovascular Medicine and Neurology, Clinical Research Institute
National Hospital Organization Kyushu Medical Center
1-8-1 Jigyohama, Chuo-ku, Fukuoka 810-8563 (Japan)
E-Mail y-okada@kyumed.jp

Uchiyama S, Amarenco P, Minematsu K, Wong KSL (eds): TIA as Acute Cerebrovascular Syndrome.
Front Neurol Neurosci. Basel, Karger, 2014, vol 33, pp 30–40 (DOI: 10.1159/000351890)

TIA Clinic: A Major Advance in Management of Transient Ischemic Attacks

Philippa Lavallée · Pierre Amarenco

INSERM U-698, Department of Neurology and Stroke Center, AP-HP, Bichat-Claude Bernard Hospital, University Paris Diderot, Sorbonne Paris Cité, Paris, France

Abstract

Patients with transient ischemic attack (TIA) are at very high risk of imminent stroke. This risk could be decreased by 80% if patients are immediately investigated and treated by stroke specialists. However, because TIA workup includes not only specialist advices but also a wide range of investigations such as brain, arterial and cardiac imaging, management of these patients in emergency required well-organized dedicated health care system, such as TIA clinics. Management of TIA patients in outpatient clinics has been shown to be safe and cost-effective avoiding full hospitalization in most of the cases.

Despite great educational efforts, stroke is still the second cause of death worldwide and is the leading cause of acquired disability. We know that the risk of stroke can be reduced by treatment of traditional vascular risk factors [1]. Among predictors of stroke, transient ischemic attack (TIA) is the most important warning sign because patients who had experienced a recent TIA are exposed to a very high risk of imminent stroke [2–4] underlining the importance of immediate assessment and treatment of these patients. Assessment of TIA patients requires diagnosis confirmation and identification of the cause in order to start effective secondary prevention to prevent a disabling vascular event. TIA identification is often difficult, and the large panel of investigations needed is nearly impossible to organize in this narrow window either for emergency department physicians in community hospital or for general practitioners (GPs), the health care providers who usually receive first call to medical attention from patients with recent TIA. Then patients are frequently sent back for outpatient investigations that will be effectively performed within one week or more. Such counterproductive pathway despite published guidelines [5–8] has several explanations; one of these is the lack of fast-track access to structure dedicated to TIA management. In the last 10 years,

TIA clinics have been developed to provide immediate access to care in case of suspicion of TIA for immediate investigations and treatment. Early experiences have shown the efficacy of such pathway by reducing the 3-month risk of stroke by 80% [9, 10].

What Is the Optimum Provision of Care in TIA Clinics?

The primary objective is to diagnose and prevent recurrent stroke and other vascular events, and educate patients on vascular risk factor management. Following AHA/ ASA, ESO and NICE guidelines [5–7], optimal TIA clinic service includes:

Fast Track Access
TIA management must not suffer any delay as the risk of recurrent stroke is high and imminent: 5% at 2 days [2], 8% at 7 days [4, 11], 7–12% at 30 days [3, 4, 11]. Hence, guidelines recommend immediate access to the TIA clinic for specialist assessment and treatment within 24 h of symptom onset for high-risk patients [8, 12, 13]. The NICE recommends that patients at a lower risk of recurrent stroke (such as patients with an $ABCD^2$ score <4) be evaluated within 48 h to one week [5]. However, 20% of patients with $ABCD^2$ score <4 have an ipsilateral >50% stenosis (either extra- or intracranial) or atrial fibrillation with a risk of recurrent stroke at 3 months, which is similar to patients with $ABCD^2$ score >4, and need to be urgently evaluated and treated [14].

Stroke Specialist Assessment
Experience always wins the day. The assessment of TIA patients by stroke specialists can positively impact their management by acting at various levels.

The first level, and probably the most obvious, is symptom recognition: Has this patient really had a TIA? In daily practice, even for stroke neurologists, accurate diagnosis of TIA remains frequently challenging [15, 16]. Transient symptoms are not synonymous with TIA and most of them can have non-ischemic origin (the so-called TIA mimics). Moreover, according to vascular territory, TIA can have a wide range of clinical presentations. If transient hemiplegia is usually not a big clinical solving issue, interpretation of subtle symptoms such as cognitive disorders, vertigo, diplopia, visual impairment, unsteadiness or dysarthria, which could occasionally be related to brain ischemia, is more difficult. Many studies have shown a poor agreement between referring physicians and stroke specialists for TIA diagnosis, with a false positivity rate as high as 60% [17, 18]. Evaluation of patients with transient neurological symptoms by stroke experts allows identifying stroke mimics avoiding unnecessary and costly investigations and therapies that could also have adverse effects.

Once the TIA diagnosis is confirmed or considered as possible, the next step is to determine which vascular territory was affected in order to guide further investigations and treatment. Correlating symptoms with the correct diseased artery is important, particularly when a carotid endarterectomy is considered because the benefit/

risk ratio for surgery is highly dependent of the presence of recent symptoms in the territory of the stenosed vessel [19]. But it is also important in order to guide the physician in the choice of arterial investigation modalities. For example, Doppler ultrasound is less sensitive for the detection of stenosis in the posterior circulation or in intracranial artery than other arterial imaging modalities such as magnetic resonance or CT angiography (MRA, CTA) [20]. Then, facing a patient with symptoms such as diplopia and vertigo, which is highly suggestive of ischemia in the posterior circulation, a stroke expert will not be reassured by a normal cervical Duplex ultrasound, and will focus further investigations on vertebral and basilar arteries.

The next step is to identify the cause in order to guide specific secondary prevention intervention. A large variety of pathological conditions can cause cerebral ischemia, and stroke subtyping requires arterial or cardiac investigations, among others. Depending on patient characteristics, clinical presentation, and clinical findings, the physician will structure and tailor the comprehensive investigation tests but also will evaluate how urgent these tests are. A left Horner's syndrome in a 40-year-old patient who recently had transient right hand numbness and left-sided cervical pain is almost pathognomonic of a left carotid dissection. In that case, detailed carotid artery imaging is absolutely required in emergency, such as axial sections of FAT-saturated MRI of the ipsilateral internal carotid artery beyond its origin that is the most sensitive tool to diagnose the arterial wall hematoma, which is specific to dissection, whereas cardiac investigations are unnecessary.

Moreover, vascular neurologists should work with a team of cardiologists and radiologists skilled in the field of stroke, knowing exactly what they have to look for and how to do it. Expertise and knowledge are undoubtedly helpful as we can see it in the daily practice, where cardiac, brain or arterial investigations are not so rarely incomplete or misinterpreted when performed by non-specialists.

Stroke specialists know the vascular and brain anatomy, both common and uncommon stroke etiologies and clinical presentations, and also general neurology to diagnose neurologic diseases that mimic stroke.

Investigations

Among the challenges of TIA management, the need of a relatively large panel of investigations is not the least. MR imaging of the brain within the first 24 h of symptom onset has become the gold standard [5–7] to diagnose cerebral infarction in case of transient focal neurologic deficit. A positive DWI allows reclassifying a TIA presentation into a cerebral infarction [21]. A negative DWI defines an actual TIA. MRI also distinguishes TIA from stroke mimics such as cerebral hemorrhage, and allows imaging of the vessels supplying the ischemic field. CT will be done if MRI is not available. ECG, 24-hour ECG monitoring, echocardiography and blood tests are usually necessary for stroke subtyping.

TIA clinics must provide, directly or via an efficient organized network, fast track access (sometimes immediate) to these different diagnostic tests needed to tailor treatment but also to help triage high-risk patients who need hospitalization for close monitoring, e.g. tight stenosis due to large artery atherosclerosis or cardiac thrombus [22], but also in less frequent disease such as non-atherosclerotic arteritis, dissection or prothrombotic states, when a specific treatment is to start without delay (e.g. endarterectomy for high grade carotid stenosis, anticoagulation in case of intracardiac thrombus). As a consequence, vascular imaging must be performed urgently, and rapid access to echocardiography (even if rarely needed in emergency) should be feasible if necessary.

Screening and treatment for vascular risk factors and coronary and/or other peripheral arterial diseases are part of services provided by TIA clinics.

Education
Education is crucial. Patients have to understand the seriousness of the disease, learn symptom recognition and what to do in case of recurrence. Importance of antithrombotic treatment and in-depth knowledge of vascular risk factors and their management are also fundamental to patient adherence and retention. A traditional outpatient GP consultation is not adapted for patient education regarding the shortness of the visit and the amount of information that has to be delivered, whereas TIA clinic environment is an ideal place to settle therapeutic educational program [23].

Network
In addition to necessary links with cardiologists and radiologists for TIA workup, TIA clinics should also facilitate access to vascular surgeon (if carotid endarterectomy is required) or endovascular therapist, but also to inpatient stroke unit if stroke unit admission is required. Telemedicine can also help diagnose TIA and guide prompt investigations in a remote area.

What Is the Ideal Setup for TIA Clinic?

Different models of service delivery have been described: outpatient setting, emergency room, dedicated hospital service for less than 24 h (day hospital). All share the same principle, according to recent guidelines [5–7]: allow TIA patients to have an urgent access to specialized stroke services. The choice between these models is largely impacted by regional, national and/or institutional differences, and, given these local specificities, are all acceptable options. No randomized trials have been performed to evaluate the benefit of TIA care provided in inpatient in comparison to outpatient settings.

Inpatient Setting
Immediate routine admission in stroke unit has been proposed as a standard care for TIA patients [24], whereas some current guidelines recommend hospitalization only for selected patients (ABCD^2 score ≥ 3; score of 0–2 and uncertainty that diagnostic

workup can be completed within 2 days as an outpatient; score of 0–2 and other evidence that indicates that patient's symptom was caused by focal ischemia) [7]. Brief hospital admission has numerous advantages. Delay for TIA assessment is eliminated (most of TIA clinics previously worked on appointment only, with recurrent strokes occurring while patients were waiting for an evaluation). Workup can be easier to perform in a short delay because all investigation tests are available on the same site. This could be particularly convenient in old patients with cognitive or walking impairment. Close monitoring of patients allows immediate thrombolysis in case of recurrent stroke. It allows continuous electrocardiogram monitoring, a useful tool for paroxysmal atrial fibrillation diagnosis but also to give treatment that could not be done in an outpatient setting (e.g. intravenous anticoagulation for cardiac valve thrombus, carotid endarterectomy). Full hospitalization is also a good opportunity to start education as more time can be dedicated to patients [25]. However, such an approach has clear limitations. The number of patients far exceeds the carrying capacity of stroke units. Hospitalization is expensive and it can also be harmful, increasing the risk of deep vein thrombosis, infections or deconditioning fragile people. The majority of patients with TIA are fit and would probably prefer not to stay in hospital if alternatives were available, improving patient satisfaction. Furthermore, if a limited number of TIA patients are at risk of imminent stroke, most of them will keep free of it. So, risk stratification is key, with low-risk patients being discharged home immediately with secondary prevention treatment prescribed.

Outpatient Setting

In 2007, a major advance in TIA management has emerged with the publication of two studies, SOS TIA [9] and EXPRESS [10] which showed that the key issue was prompt assessment and treatment by stroke specialists in a dedicated clinic. Moreover, they showed this could be done safely on an outpatient setting basis. Patients were referred to the clinic by GPs in EXPRESS and by physicians or emergency departments in SOS TIA. Assessment was immediate (after a brief phone interview of the referring doctor) – 24 h a day/7 days a week in SOS TIA, and semi urgent (without contact with referring physician) – every weekday afternoon in EXPRESS. In both studies, the median delay from seeking first medical attention in primary care to assessment in TIA clinic was less than one day. Workup was performed rapidly in both studies but was slightly different. In EXPRESS, brain imaging was performed in the case of incomplete resolution of symptoms, EKG was systematically performed on the same day, echocardiography (only when clinically indicated) and carotid ultrasound were arranged during the following week (neither the rate of investigation testing nor the definition of clinical relevance was available). In SOS TIA, all patients with confirmed or possible TIA diagnosis after stroke specialist assessment had a same day standardized workup including brain imaging (mostly CT scan during the 2003–2007 period of this study), EKG, cervical duplex and transcranial Doppler ultrasonography and blood tests. Urgent echocardiography was performed only if a high risk of recurrent embolism from cardiac source was suspected (e.g. endocarditis, prosthetic valve thrombosis). A second set of investigations was planned with MRI, MRA, and echocardiography. In total, 95% of the patients had brain imaging, arterial and cardiac investigations. Antithrombotic treatment was started immediately in both studies. In EXPRESS, simvastatin and blood pressure-lowering drugs (if no contraindication) were added on the same day. In SOS TIA, vascular risk factor management could be either added immediately in a second visit or sometimes only recommendations were made to the referring physicians. This standard of care based on the simple idea of urgent specialized assessment and early initiation of existing treatment was associated with an 80% reduction in the risk of early recurrent stroke. Since then, different models of organization, all based on acute management and treatment by specialists, have been proposed to expedite the acute management of TIA patient as outpatients with a similar rate of stroke. Several are built on the same model described in SOS TIA and EXPRESS [26, 27], whereas others did not use a dedicated clinic but an urgent evaluation in the emergency department by a stroke specialist [28].

If there is no doubt that the outpatient setting is feasible, safe and effective, inevitably some patients (mainly those at higher risk of stroke but also for cardiac monitoring or patient convenience) will need to be hospitalized. In SOS TIA, the first set of investigations was also used as a triage system for full hospital admission decision-making (high risk of recurrence, cardiac monitoring, patient convenience). In this study, 25% of the patients (18% in EXPRESS Study) were admitted to the stroke unit, which was easy to organize because the clinic was set within a comprehensive stroke center that included both the TIA clinic and the stroke unit with an intensive care unit available 24 h a day/7 days a week.

Opening outpatient TIA clinics in a stroke unit (such as the SOS TIA setup) is probably a good way to improve the provision of care, to share human and material resources in order to reduce costs and to make possible immediate hospitalization only if necessary.

Preadmission Triage for TIA Clinic Appointment

Considering that local resources are frequently insufficient to provide immediate access to appropriate structure for all TIA patients and that the vast majority of patients with suspicion of TIA will not experience a recurrent stroke in the next 3 months because the underlying cause is not at high risk of recurrence or because the transient neurologic symptoms were not of ischemic origin, preadmission triage tools have been developed and are currently used to select patients at higher risk of stroke for urgent versus delayed appointment in TIA clinics.

Regarding the high proportion of patients with definite non-cerebrovascular diagnosis sent by community physicians in TIA clinics [17, 18], the first line of triage should concern 'positive diagnosis' in order to detect patients with evident non-ischemic symptoms but also patients with symptoms in evolution who could be eligible for thrombolysis. Telephone hotline, dedicated to community primary care physicians, with immediate access to stroke specialist assistance has been proposed to triage the patients on the basis of all available information [9, 29]. Community primary care physicians were informed of the opening of the hotline by mail [9–29] and email [29]. In the SOS-TIA experience, an educational leaflet with clear guidelines was sent at the same time to 15,000 community primary care physicians and specialists that may see TIA patients seeking first medical attention. In the SOS TIA clinic experience, patients with non-ischemic symptoms accounted for only 22% of all admissions to the clinic [9]. In the Scottish experience, 94% of the referring physicians were very satisfied with the hotline services, and the additional workload related to phone call for stroke specialists was about 40 min each weekday (80% of the calls occurred during week days between 9 a.m. and 5 p.m.) for a hotline covering a population of 800,000 [29]. Besides patient triage, live interaction with referring physicians could also help stroke specialists to anticipate patient admission if considering patient history, hospital admission or special investigations will be required.

Because at 2 days 95% of the patients with a suspicion of TIA will remain free of symptoms, investigators have developed risk stratification tools (described in detail in a dedicated chapter) to triage patients at higher risk of imminent stroke in order to assist physicians in making decisions regarding urgency of investigations or hospital admission. The 7-point $ABCD^2$ clinical score has been incorporated in some guidelines [5, 8], which required semi-urgent investigations (within 48 h to one week) for patients with a score <4 or urgent investigations (within 24 h) for a score ≥4 and for patients with crescendo TIA [5, 8] or with non-anticoagulated atrial fibrillation [8]. Such clinical scores have clear limitations. First, it has been shown that the $ABCD^2$ is less accurate when calculated by a non-stroke physician [20–31], a finding that raises concerns as the score has been designed to be used by primary care non-specialist physicians for TIA triage. Second, and most importantly, the $ABCD^2$ score is blinded to stroke etiology, whereas stroke cause/mechanism largely drives the risk of subsequent stroke and the choice of preventive treatment. In the SOS TIA cohort, 20% of the patients with an $ABCD^2$ score <4 had symptomatic large arterial atherosclerosis stenosis >50% or a major cardiac source of embolism [32], and among TIA patients with an $ABCD^2$ score <4, those having symptomatic large arterial atherosclerosis stenosis >50% or a major cardiac source of embolism had a 90-day stroke risk similar to patients with TIA with an $ABCD^2$ score ≥4 [33]. Due to the nature of its components (older age, high blood pressure, presence of diabetes, presence of motor deficit or speech impairment), the $ABCD^2$ score will be more prone to identify TIA related to large-artery atherosclerosis or atrial fibrillation (stroke causes at high risk of recurrence) but will probably be less efficient in correctly grading risk patients with rarest disease also at high risk of stroke recurrence but not related to traditional risk factors (e.g. dissection, mitral stenosis, endocarditis…) or with vertebrobasilar TIA. For the same reason, patients with low $ABCD^2$ score have more chance to have stroke mimics than true TIA as suggested by several studies [34, 35]. Now, several updated versions of the $ABCD^2$ score have been proposed adding items for advanced etiologic subtyping and positive brain MRI diffusion that improves stroke risk prediction [36, 37]. However, the need for a larger range of investigations diminishes the original purpose of the $ABCD^2$ score as a simple clinical tool to stratify risk in TIA patients and renders the concept of risk stratification for primary care physicians meaningless. In conclusion, due to the pitfalls of clinical score risk, once identified as a possible TIA, and once possible, patients should be evaluated without delay regardless of $ABCD^2$ score.

Finally, triage tools would be helpful to identify those patients who will benefit from hospitalization instead of outpatient care because they are at high risk of recurrence or because it increases the chance to find out paroxysmal atrial fibrillation. For patients with identified cause at high risk of recurrence after quick diagnostic evaluation (e.g. large arterial high-grade stenosis, cardiac disease at high risk of embolism), hospitalization is recommended. However, uncertainties remain for patients with initial negative workup and $ABCD^2$ score ≥4 and also for those with an ischemic lesion on DWI MRI who seem to be at higher risk of recurrent stroke [33, 36, 37]. Whether those patients will benefit from hospitalization deserves further research.

Are TIA Clinics Cost-Effective?

There are very few data on the costs of TIA clinics. Further analysis of the EXPRESS study has shown that urgent versus delayed assessment of patients with TIA or minor stroke in an outpatient TIA clinic significantly reduced subsequent hospital bed-days by 4, a reduction driven by reduction in days in hospital due to recurrent stroke, allowing a cost saving of GBP 624 per patient referred to the clinic [38]. A recent study using decision modeling techniques has evaluated the short-term and long-term cost-effectiveness of hospitalization versus urgent outpatient clinic referral in patients presenting with TIA. They found that hospital-based hospitalization was cost-prohibitive with an additional cost of USD 5,573 per patient [39].

Conclusion

It is now obvious that TIA patients require immediate assessment and treatment by stroke specialists. By providing a fast-track access to stroke experts and to appropriate investigations including brain, arterial and cardiac investigations, and emergent treatment, TIA clinics have shown to be highly effective in the prevention of stroke recurrence. Systematic hospitalization is not necessary, and outpatient TIA clinics have proved to be safe and probably cost effective. Identification of high-risk patients requiring hospitalization remains challenging. But quick triage based on identification of causes at high risk of recurrence such as large arterial high-grade stenosis, evidence of cardiac embolism or less frequent but worrisome causes (arteritis, dissection) is feasible and helpful. Uncertainties remain for patients with negative or not clinically relevant finding after a minimal workup and an ABCD^2 score ≥4 which carry a 3% stroke risk [33], and for those with a recent ischemic lesion on DWI MRI. The main limitation of TIA clinics is the limited resources available. More than two decades ago, efforts were made to improve stroke care with the generalization of stroke units. Those departments are the ideal setup to accommodate outpatient TIA clinics. It is now up to the various health authorities and other academic institutions to include the presence of outpatient TIA clinics in the specifications for 'comprehensive' stroke unit. Finally, efforts should be made to improve public education as general awareness of TIA symptoms and the need to seek medical attention urgently remain poor [40].

References

1 Hackam DG, Spence JD: Combining multiple approaches for the secondary prevention of vascular events after stroke. Stroke 2007;38:1881–1885.
2 Johnston SC, Gress DR, Browner WS, Sidney S: Short-term prognosis after emergency department diagnosis of TIA. JAMA 2000;284:2901–2906.
3 Hill MD, Yiannakoulias N, Jeerakathil T, Tu JV, Svenson LW, Schopflocher DP: The high risk of stroke immediately after transient ischemic attack: a population-based study. Neurology 2004;62:2015–2020.
4 Coull A, Lovett JK, Rothwell PM, the Oxford Vascular Study: Early risk of stroke after a TIA or minor stroke in a population-based incidence study. BMJ 2004;328:326–328.
5 National Institute for Health and Clinical Excellence: NICE clinical guideline 68. Stroke: diagnosis and initial management of acute stroke and transient ischaemic attack (TIA). July 2008. http://www. nice. org.uk/CG068 (accessed June 28, 2011).
6 ESO Guidelines for Management of Ischaemic Stroke 2008.
7 Easton JD, Saver JL, Albers GW, Alberts MJ, Chaturvedi S, Feldmann E, Hatsukami TS, Higashida RT, Johnston SC, Kidwell CS, Lutsep HL, Miller E, Sacco RL: Definition and evaluation of transient ischemic attack: a scientific statement for healthcare professionals from the American Heart Association/American Stroke Association Stroke Council; Council on Cardiovascular Surgery and Anesthesia; Council on Cardiovascular Radiology and Intervention; Council on Cardiovascular Nursing; and the Interdisciplinary Council on Peripheral Vascular Disease: The American Academy of Neurology affirms the value of this statement as an educational tool for neurologists. Stroke 2009;40:2276–2293.
8 National Institute of Clinical Studies: Emergency department stroke and transient ischaemic attack care bundle: information and implementation package. Melbourne, National Health and Medical Research Council, 2009.
9 Lavallee PC, Meseguer E, Abboud H, Cabrejo L, Olivot JM, Simon O, Mazighi M, Nifle C, Niclot P, Lapergue B, Klein IF, Brochet E, Steg OG, Leseche G, Labreuche J, Touboul PJ, Amerenco P: A transient ischaemic attack clinic with round-the-clock access (SOS-TIA): feasibility and effects. Lancet Neurol 2007;6:953–960.
10 Rothwell PM, Eliasziw M, Gutnikov SA, Warlow CP, Barnett HJM: Endarterectomy for symptomatic carotid stenosis in relation to clinical subgroups and timing of surgery. Lancet 2004;363:915–924.
11 Lovett J, Dennis M, Sandercock PAG, Bamford J, Warlow CP, Rothwell PM: The very early risk of stroke following a TIA. Stroke 2003;34:e138–e140.
12 ANAES: Prise en charge diagnostique et traitement immédiat de l'accident ischémique transitoire de l'adulte. Recommandations pour la pratique clinique, mai 2004. www.anaes.fr.
13 National Collaborating Center for chronic conditions: Stroke: National Clinical Guidelines for diagnosis and initial management of acute stroke and transient ischemic attack (TIA). London, Royal College of Physicians, 2008.
14 Amarenco P, Julien Labreuche J, Lavallee PC: Patients with transient ischemic attack with ABCD2 <4 can have similar 90-day stroke risk as patients with transient ischemic attack with ABCD2 >4. Stroke 2012;43:863–865.

15 Castle J, Mlynash M, Lee K, et al: Agreement regarding diagnosis of transient ischemic attack fairly low among stroke-trained neurologists. Stroke 2010;41: 1367–1370.
16 Kraaijeveld CL, van Gijn J, Schouten HJ, Staal A: Interobserver agreement for the diagnosis of transient ischemic attacks. Stroke 1984;15:723–725.
17 Dennis MS, Bamford JM, Sandercock PA, Warlow CP: Incidence of transient ischemic attacks in Oxfordshire, England. Stroke 1989;20:333–339.
18 Prabhakaran S, Silver AJ, Warrior L, McClenathan B, Lee VH: Misdiagnosis of transient ischemic attacks in the emergency room. Cerebrovasc Dis 2008;26: 630–635.
19 Rothwell PM, Eliasziw M, Gutnikov SA, Warlow CP, Barnett HJM, the Carotid Endarterectomy Trialists' Collaboration: Endarterectomy for symptomatic carotid stenosis in relation to clinical subgroups and timing of surgery. Lancet 2004;363: 915–924.
20 Khan S, Cloud GC, Kerry S, Markus HS: Imaging of vertebral artery stenosis: a systematic review. J Neurol Neurosurg Psychiatry 2007;78:1218–1225.
21 Albers GW, Caplan LR, Easton JD, Fayad PB, Mohr JP, Saver JL, Sherman DG, TIA Working Group. Transient ischemic attack, proposal for a new definition. N Engl J Med 2002;347:1713–1716.
22 Purroy F, Montaner J, Molina CA, Pilar Delgado P, Ribo M, Alvarez-Sabín J: Patterns and predictors of early risk of recurrence after transient ischemic attack with respect to etiologic subtypes. Stroke 2007; 38:3225–3229.
23 Mouradian MS, Hussain MS, Lari H, Salam A, Senthilselvan A, Dean N, Shuaib A: The impact of a stroke prevention clinic in diagnosing modifiable risk factors for stroke. Can J Neurol Sci 2005;32:496–500.
24 Walter A, Seidel G, Thie A, Raspe H: Semi-intensive stroke unit versus conventional care in acute ischemic stroke or TIA: a prospective study in Germany. J Neurol Sci 2009;287:131–137.
25 Touze E, Coste J, Voicu M, et al: Importance of in-hospital initiation of therapies and therapeutic inertia in secondary stroke prevention: Implementation of Prevention After a Cerebrovascular evenT (IMPACT) Study. Stroke 2008;39:1834–1843.
26 Wasserman J, Perry J, Dowlatshahi D, Stotts G, Stiell I, Sutherland J, Symington C, Sharma M: Stratified urgent care for transient ischemic attack results in low stroke rates. Stroke 2010;41:2601–2605.
27 Olivot JM, Wolford C, Castle J, Mlynash M, Schwartz NE, Lansberg MG, Kemp S, Albers GW: TWO ACES: Transient ischemic attack work-up as outpatient assessment of clinical evaluation and safety. Stroke 2011;42:1839–1843.
28 Kim AS, Sidney S, Bernstein AL, Douglas VC, Johnston SC: Urgent neurology consultation from the ED for transient ischemic attack. Am J Emerg Med 2011; 29:601–608.
29 Kerr E, Arulraj N, Scott M, McDowall M, van Dijke M, Keir S, Sandercock P, Dennis M: A telephone hotline for transient ischaemic attack and stroke: prospective audit of a model to improve rapid access to specialist stroke care. BMJ 2010; 341:c3265.
30 Perry JJ, Sharma M, Sivilotti ML, Sutherland J, Symington C, Worster A, Émond M, Stotts G, Jin AY, Oczkowski WJ, Sahlas DJ, Murray HE, MacKey A, Verreault S, Wells GA, Stiell IG, et al: Prospective validation of the ABCD2 score for patients in the emergency department with transient ischemic attack. CMAJ 2011;183:1137–1145.
31 Sanders LM, Srikanth VK, Blacker DJ, Jolley DJ, Cooper KA, Phan TG: Performance of the ABCD2 score for stroke risk post TIA: meta-analysis and probability modeling. Neurology 2012;79: 971–980.
32 Amarenco P, Julien Labreuche J, Lavallee PC, Meseguer E, Cabrejo L, Slaoui T, Guidoux C, Olivot JM, Abboud H, Lapergue B, Klein IF, Mazighi M, Touboul PJ: Does ABCD2 score below 4 allow more time to evaluate patients with a transient ischemic attack? Stroke 2009;40:3091–3095.
33 Amarenco P, Julien Labreuche J, Lavallee PC: Patients with transient ischemic attack with ABCD2 <4 can have similar 90-day stroke risk as patients with transient ischemic attack with ABCD2 >4. Stroke 2012;43:863–865.
34 Josephson SA, Sidney S, Pham TN, Bernstein AL, Johnston SC: Higher ABCD2 score predicts patients most likely to have true transient ischemic attack. Stroke 2008;39:3096–3098.
35 Sheehan OC, Merwick A, Kelly LA, Hannon N, Marnane M, Kyne L, et al: Diagnostic usefulness of the ABCD2 score to distinguish transient ischemic attack and minor ischemic stroke from noncerebrovascular events: the North Dublin TIA Study. Stroke 2009;40:3449–3454.
36 Merwick A, Albers GW, Amarenco P, Arsava EM, Ay H, Calvet D, Coutts SB, Cucchiara BL, Demchuk AM, Furie KL, Giles MF, Labreuche J, Lavallée PC, Mas JL, Olivot JM, Purroy F, Rothwell PM, Saver JL, Sheehan ÓC, Stack JP, Walsh C, Kelly PJ: Addition of brain and carotid imaging to the ABCD score to identify patients at early risk of stroke after transient ischaemic attack: a multicentre observational study. Lancet Neurol 2010;9: 1060–1069.

37 Engelter ST, Amort M, Jax F, Weisskopf F, Katan M, Burow A, Bonati LH, Hatz F, Wetzel FG, Fluri F, Lyrer PA: Optimizing the risk estimation after a transient ischaemic attack: the ABCDE plus sign in circle score. Eur J Neurol 2012;19:55–61.
38 Luengo-Fernandez R, Gray AM, Rothwell PM: Effect of urgent treatment for transient ischaemic attack and minor stroke on disability and hospital costs (EXPRESS study): a prospective population-based sequential comparison. Lancet Neurol 2009;8:235–243.
39 Joshi JK, Ouyang B, Prabhakaran S: Should TIA patients be hospitalized or referred to a same-day clinic? A decision analysis. Neurology 2011;77:2082–2088.
40 Johnston SC, Fayad PB, Gorelick PB, Hanley DF, Shwayder P, van Husen D, Weiskopf T: Prevalence and knowledge of transient ischemic attack among US adults. Neurology 2003;60:1429–1434.

Prof. Pierre Amarenco
Department of Neurology and Stroke Centre, AP-HP, Bichat-Claude Bernard Hospital
University Paris Diderot, Sorbonne Paris Cité, INSERM U698
46, rue Henri Huchard, FR–75018 Paris (France)
E-Mail pierre.amarenco@bch.aphp.fr

Uchiyama S, Amarenco P, Minematsu K, Wong KSL (eds): TIA as Acute Cerebrovascular Syndrome.
Front Neurol Neurosci. Basel, Karger, 2014, vol 33, pp 41–68 (DOI: 10.1159/000351891)

Risk Scores for Transient Ischemic Attack

M.E. Wolf · V.E. Held · M.G. Hennerici

Department of Neurology, UniversitätsMedizin Mannheim UMM, University of Heidelberg, Mannheim, Germany

Abstract

The risk of recurrent ischemic stroke after a transient ischemic attack (TIA) has been reported to be 5–10%, and is elevated especially within the first days after the index event. Since TIA primarily has a good outcome without persisting new deficits, interest has been growing to predict stroke recurrence after TIA. This has led to the development of scores, initially for long-term prognosis such as the Stroke Prognosis Instrument (SPI) or the Hankey score, which both have shown a good predictive value at 1 or 2 years after TIA. Risk factors such as age, hypertension or cardiovascular disease were integrated in these systems. Since the early risk prediction for stroke in patients presenting within 24 h after onset of symptoms became clinically more and more relevant in emergency stroke units, the ABCD score (for the predictive factors Age, Blood pressure, Clinical symptoms, Duration of symptoms) was developed. Validation was promising, and hence further scores were developed, which entailed a large number of studies trying to validate these systems or to improve them (e.g. $ABCD^2$, $ABCD^2$I, $ABCD^3$, $ABCD^3$I, CIP model, ASPIRE approach, ABCDE+ etc.). The main approaches were to include imaging results (such as DWI positivity) or etiologic considerations (e.g. carotid stenosis or atrial fibrillation). However, these new scores necessitate an extensive diagnostic workup, and therefore can only be used in large stroke centers. Currently, for acute TIA management, the use of $ABCD^2$ is recommended in several guidelines.

The risk of recurrent ischemic stroke after a transient ischemic attack (TIA) has been reported to be 5–10% [1]. Especially within the first days after the index event, a high percentage of recurrent neurologic symptoms has been reported [2]. Correspondingly, 15% of patients suffering from ischemic stroke report previous TIA [3], and the prevalence of TIA preceding ischemic stroke (anamnestic details and information of chronic ischemic lesions on MRI) has been estimated at >20% in some studies [2].

Due to the transient character of neurologic symptoms in TIA, the neurologic outcome of patients seems favorable. However, with the elevated risk of early recurrent ischemic stroke, TIA must be considered a warning sign for an unfavorable course. Therefore, a complete stroke workup after TIA should be performed to detect potential etiologies (e.g. atrial fibrillation (AF) or carotid stenosis), which can be treated immediately to prevent major ischemic stroke in the further course.

Since subsequent stroke might occur within 24 h after TIA, there is a need to early identify patients with a risk to develop ischemic stroke because they need a full workup and/or treatment and therefore necessarily hospitalization. A distinction between TIA patients needing acute diagnostic workup in hospital and TIA patients who can be further evaluated in an outpatient clinic would permit a patient-adapted workflow, sparing some patients an unnecessary long stay at hospital while providing a secure stay at hospital for high-risk patients. Additionally, in a time period when economic constraints become more and more important, the risk- and cost-benefit relation could be optimized in this way.

These notions have led to several attempts to stratify the risk of stroke after a first TIA by creating risk scores and application of these to validate the screening tool. In the closely related specialty of cardiology, the Framingham Score has shown good results and usefulness of such a score, in this particular case for detection of coronary heart disease [4]. Therefore, the idea was to find a similar scoring system to identify TIA patients with a high risk for recurrent stroke.

The idea to build a score needs many variables to consider before developing a useful tool. A good score should include characteristics such as [5] predictive value and consistency of performance (in different studies with different settings), and the score should be easy to calculate for daily use in emergency room situations.

It is important to know that the risk estimation also depends on the clinical specialty of the physician (e.g. a general practitioner or a specialized stroke neurologist) and the setting of evaluation (e.g. emergency room or TIA clinic), which therefore influence the results of validation. Finally, the method of data extraction might bias the results as well.

Several attempts have been made since the 1990s, somehow with different points of view or interests. Scores could be divided into short-time risk of recurrent stroke versus middle- or long-time risk [6]. Another classification could differentiate between scores with only clinical information versus scores including complementary investigations: scores for TIA only, or TIA and minor stroke, or even risk of stroke after TIA versus the prediction of a first stroke or TIA based on clinical information. In this chapter, however, we would like to take a sequential approach, describing consecutive developments of different scores, since this might best reflect the dynamics and growing importance of such a system in stroke neurology.

Chapters will be organized into 3 paragraphs: '*Background*' will shortly explain the aim of the study or development of the score in its time, '*Definition of the System*' will follow for the reader, who wants a quick overlook. In the '*Validation*' paragraph, the development of the score (which might be the basis for the '*Definition*' paragraph) and further evaluation and application of the score are discussed.

Risk of Recurrent Stroke after Transient Ischemic Attack

The history of risk score developments can be divided into two main aspects: evaluation of *long-term* risk for stroke, which coincides with the time period in the 1990s, and evaluation of *short-time* prognosis, which was focused on in the 2000s. In consequence, we divided this chapter into these two parts.

Subsequently, we chose to show the most important results in our opinion to provide a best available comprehensive presentation and tried to generate a systematic overview despite the heterogeneous data due to different designs, populations, and outcome parameters in the performed studies. Table 1 summarizes the scores with their definitions and risk group assessment.

First Long-Term Approaches: Stroke Prognosis Instrument I/II and Hankey Score, etc.

Stroke Prognosis Instrument I (SPI-I) [7]

Background

The SPI was developed for patients with transient ischemia or minor ischemic stroke in the vascular territory of the internal carotid artery. Patients had no previous cerebrovascular event; patients with an artificial heart valve were excluded. The focus on the anterior circulation was due to the special interest of the investigators in carotid artery morphology.

Definition of the System

The initial SPI prognostic system used three parameters to define risk groups: age >65 years (3 points); diabetes mellitus (3 points); arterial hypertension (2 points). Arterial hypertension was defined using measurements on day 1–3 at hospital and categorized as follows: severe hypertension >180/100 mm Hg (on 2 days); no hypertension <170/94 mm Hg (not higher at ≥1 day); mild hypertension between 'severe' and 'no' hypertension. Potential risk groups were defined as follows: risk group 1: 0 points; risk group 2: 1–5 points; risk group 3: 6–8 points.

The initial study to validate these factors led to a modified SPI, defined as the final SPI-I. Coronary heart disease (1 point) and the distinction between stroke and TIA for baseline event (2 points for stroke) were integrated ending up in the following sys-

Table 1. Risk scores for TIA (some for TIA and minor stroke) to predict the recurrence of stroke after TIA (detailed explanations are given in the corresponding paragraphs)

Score/study	Considered risk factors/parameters	Scoring system: distribution of points; subdivision of risk groups
SPI-I [7]	Age >65 years Diabetes Severe hypertension >180/100 mm Hg Coronary artery disease Distinction between stroke and TIA for baseline event (stroke)	3 points 3 points 2 points 1 point 2 points Maximum score: 11 Risk group 1: 0–2 points Risk group 2: 3–6 points Risk group 3: 7–11 points
Hankey score [10]	Age Female Amaurosis fugax Carotid and vertebrobasilar TIAs More than 1 TIA in the last 3 months Peripheral vascular disease Left ventricular hypertrophy (ECG) Residual neurological signs	Complex equation, calculating the probability of stroke-free survival at 1 and 5 years after TIA (see corresponding paragraph)
SPI–II [9]	Age >70 years Diabetes Hypertension >180/100 mm Hg Coronary artery disease Distinction between stroke and TIA for baseline event (stroke) Congestive heart failure Prior stroke	2 points 3 points 1 point 1 point 2 points 3 points 3 points Maximum score: 15 Risk group 1: 0–3 points Risk group 2: 4–7 points Risk group 3: 8–15 points
LiLAC [17]	Age Male sex Diabetes mellitus Peripheral arterial disease Index event stroke vs. TIA Paresis Dysarthria	Calculation of hazard ratios and further processing with a complex formula
ESRS [14]	Age 65–75 years Age >75 years Arterial hypertension Diabetes mellitus Previous MI Other cardiovascular disease (except MI and atrial fibrillation)	1 point 2 points 1 point 1 point 1 point 1 point

Table 1. Continued

Score/study	Considered risk factors/parameters	Scoring system: distribution of points; subdivision of risk groups
	Peripheral arterial disease (PAD)	1 point
	Smoker	1 point
	Previous TIA or ischemic stroke in addition to qualifying event	1 point
		Maximum score: 9 points
		Low risk 0–2 points
		Higher risk ≥3 points
California Risk Score [22]	Age ≥60 years	1 point
	Diabetes	1 point
	Unilateral weakness	1 point
	Speech impairment	1 point
	Symptom duration >10 min	1 point
		Maximum score: 5
ABCD [6]	Age ≥60 years	1 point
	Blood pressure ≥140/90 mm Hg	1 point
	Clinical features	
	Unilateral weakness	2 points
	Speech disturbance without weakness	1 point
	Other	0 points
	Duration of symptoms	
	≥60 min	2 points
	10–59 min	1 point
	<10 min	0 points
		Maximum score: 6
		Low risk ≤3
		Intermediate to high risk >3
ABCD^2 [25]		
	Age ≥60 years	1 point
	Blood pressure ≥140/90 mm Hg	1 point
	Clinical features	
	Unilateral weakness	2 points
	Speech impairment without weakness	1 point
	Duration of symptoms	
	≥60 min	2 points
	10–59 min	1 point
	Diabetes	1 point
		Maximum score: 7
		Low risk <4
		Intermediate risk 4–5
		High risk >5
ABCD^2 + MRI [47]	Age ≥60 years	1 point
	Blood pressure ≥140/90 mm Hg	1 point
	Clinical features	
	Unilateral weakness	2 points
	Speech impairment without weakness	1 point

Table 1. Continued

Score/study	Considered risk factors/parameters	Scoring system: distribution of points; subdivision of risk groups
	Duration of symptoms	
	≥60 min	2 points
	10–59 min	1 point
	Diabetes	1 point
	MRI lesion (DWI positive or mismatch)	1 point
	Evidence of intracranial vessel occlusion	1 point
		Maximum score: 9 Low risk 0–4 Intermediate risk 5–6 High risk 7–9
Clinical and Imaging-based prediction model: CIP-model [34]	$ABCD^2$ stratification + consideration of DWI positivity on MRI	Low risk: DWI negative High risk: DWI positive or $ABCD^2$ ≥4 + DWI positive
$ABCD^2$-I [35]	Age ≥60 years	1 point
	Blood pressure ≥140/90 mm Hg	1 point
	Clinical features	
	Unilateral weakness	2 points
	Speech impairment without weakness	1 point
	Duration of symptoms	
	≥60 min	2 points
	10–59 min	1 point
	Diabetes	1 point
	Brain infarction on imaging	3 points
		Maximum score: 10
$ABCD^3$ [36]	Age ≥60 years	1 point
	Blood pressure ≥140/90 mm Hg	1 point
	Clinical features	
	Unilateral weakness	2 points
	Speech impairment without weakness	1 point
	Duration of symptoms	
	≥60 min	2 points
	10–59 min	1 point
	Diabetes	1 point
	Prior TIA within 1 week	2 points
		Maximum score: 9 Low risk 0–3 Intermediate risk 4–5 High risk 6–9
$ABCD^3$-I [36]	Age ≥60 years	1 point
	Blood pressure ≥140/90 mm Hg	1 point
	Clinical features	
	Unilateral weakness	2 points
	Speech impairment without weakness	1 point
	Duration of symptoms	
	≥60 min	2 points
	10–59 min	1 point

Table 1. Continued

Score/study	Considered risk factors/parameters	Scoring system: distribution of points; subdivision of risk groups
	Diabetes	1 point
	Prior TIA within 1 week	2 points
	Stenosis on carotid imaging (≥50%)	2 points
	Abnormal DWI	2 points
		Maximum score: 13
		Low risk 0–3
		Intermediate risk 4–7
		High risk 8–13
ASPIRE approach [39]	ABCD^2 score ≥4 OR	Considered as high risk
	Motor/speech symptoms lasting >5 min OR	
	Atrial fibrillation	
ABCDE+ [40]	Age ≥60 years	1 point
	Blood pressure ≥140/90 mm Hg	1 point
	Clinical features	
	Unilateral weakness	2 points
	Speech impairment without weakness	1 point
	Duration of symptoms	
	≥60 min	2 points
	10–59 min	1 point
	Diabetes	1 point
	Etiology	
	Large artery atherosclerosis	3 points
	Cardioembolism	1 point
	Undetermined	1 point
	Small vessel disease	0 points
	Other	0 points
	DWI positive	3 points
		Maximum score: 13
		Low risk ≤6
		High risk >6

tem: age >65 years (3 points); diabetes (3 points); hypertension (2 points); coronary heart disease (1 point); distinction between stroke and TIA for baseline event (2 points for stroke). Risk groups were divided into risk group 1: 0–2 points; risk group 2: 3–6 points and risk group 3: 7–11 points. Table 1 gives an overview of all scores with their definition and risk group assessment.

Validation of the System/Studies

The initial validation [7] included 142 patients (Yale cohort). The study end point was stroke or death within 2 years and was reached in 27%. Of these 55% had a stroke, 11% had a stroke and died and 34% died without having a stroke. While bivariate analysis showed a relative risk (RR) in 4 potential predictive categories [age >65 years (RR 2.4); diabetes mellitus (RR 2, 4); female gender (RR 1.7); severe hypertension (RR 1.8)], a stepwise proportional hazard model only detected the 3 variables which were used for the scoring system [age >65 years (RR 2.55); diabetes mellitus (RR 2.78); severe hypertension (RR 1.92)]. Analyzing the outcome according to the risk groups, a significant difference was found ($p < 0.001$) with a reached end point in 2% of group 1, 31% of group 2 and 54% of group 3.

In addition, the data of the Canadian Cooperative Study group [8] were analyzed as a second independent cohort (330 patients; slightly modified definitions of arterial hypertension and coronary heart disease due to the data available). The risk group splitting was useful again (end point in group 1 in 12%, group 2 in 21%, group 3 in 31%; $p < 0.04$), but not as impressive as with the Yale cohort.

Further analysis of the Canadian cohort helped to identify 5 predictors [distinction between stroke and TIA for baseline event (RR for minor stroke 2.7); age >65 years (RR 1.8); previous episode of transient ischemia or stroke (RR 1.8); severe hypertension (RR 1.8); coronary heart disease (RR 1.7)]. Since the initial scoring system only considered 2 of these, the modified, final SPI-I score was created, as defined above. Final analysis with the SPI-I showed promising results for both cohorts (end point reached in Yale cohort/Canadian cohort: group 1: 3/10%; group 2: 27/21%; group 3: 48/59%).

Further validation was performed in 4 independent cohorts in the context of the development of Stroke Prognosis Instrument II (SPI-II) [9]. In summary, the pooled analysis revealed a risk for stroke or death within 2 years after TIA or minor stroke of 9, 17 and 24% ($p < 0.01$), respectively, for risk groups 1–3, therefore confirming a valid discrimination of risk groups with this system.

Hankey Score [10]

Background

The aim was to develop a prediction model for major vascular outcome events in patients with TIA to identify the patients with a high risk for major stroke after TIA. The retrospective character of SPI-I studies and the small sample size had been criticized; therefore, the authors chose a prospective approach.

Definition of the System

In a complex stepwise approach, significantly relevant risk factors were identified in a first step and further analyzed with multiple regression analysis, leading to a prediction model of absolute stroke risk. Predictive models for the 3 outcome parameters (stroke, coronary event or stroke/myocardial infarction, MI/vascular death) of the study were defined. The predictive equation for survival free of stroke reads as follows:

START		
Age–60	Multiplied by	4.5
Female	Subtract	36
Amaurosis fugax only	Subtract	72
Carotid and vertebrobasilar TIAs	Add	53
More than 1 TIA in the last 3 months	Add	[1.6 × (n – 1)]
Peripheral vascular disease	Add	76
Left ventricular hypertrophy (ECG)	Add	68
Residual neurological signs	Add	74
	=	Total cumulative score 'y'
Divide 'y' by 100 and exponentiate $e^{(y/100)}$	=	'x'

The probability of survival free of stroke can then be calculated:
At 1 year = 0.96^x
At 5 years = 0.88^x

Validation of the System/Studies

In the initial study [10], 469 TIA patients (with a presumed etiology of large vessel disease, small vessel disease or cardioembolism) were followed up over a median of 4.1 years. Outcome events were stroke, coronary event or stroke/MI/vascular death (whichever occurred first). Stroke occurred in 63 patients, 58 had a coronary event, 118 suffered a stroke/MI/vascular death. The stepwise analysis of detected prognostic factors for stroke such as increasing age, male sex, increasing number of TIAs in the months before presentation, peripheral vascular disease, ischemic heart disease and TIAs of the brain (compared with the eye) led to the equation which is explained above. Interestingly, carotid stenosis was found to be a highly significant factor for recurrent stroke, but did not increase the power of the algorithm and therefore is not part of the final equation.

After the original publication, the Hankey score was tested in an independent population-based cohort of 1,653 TIA patients in the UK-TIA aspirin trial and 107 TIA patients in the Oxfordshire Community Stroke Project [11]. The aim was to test the reliability of prediction (group analysis) and the ability to discriminate between patients with low and high risk (individual analysis) using this system. The reliability of the equations showed promising results for lower risk patients (defined as 0–30% of risk for one of the 3 outcome events within 5 years), but for higher risk patients (>30–40% of risk) an overestimation was observed. The discrimination between patients with low and high risk for recurrent stroke remained complicated since there is no single important prognostic factor which could indicate the risk. The authors of the study concluded that the algorithm is useful to reliably estimate the absolute 5-year risk of a serious vascular event, but that a differentiation between low-risk and high-risk patients is not possible with this system. The authors recommended an arbitrary cutoff at 30% of risk for an outcome event at 5 years. As a general observation, most of the outcome events occurred in TIA patients with a low risk profile, underlining the difficulties of classifying patients as low risk. Further validation with the data of the Dutch TIA Trial (DTT) and the ECST trial was planned, but no publication was found.

SPI-II [9]

Background
Since some criticism of SPI-I had been expressed, the authors of the SPI-I started an additional attempt to (a) validate the SPI-I in 4 independent cohorts and (b) identify new additional predictive values, which were integrated in an improved scoring system named SPI-II.

Definition of the System
The main modifications compared with the SPI-I were a modification of the age as predictive factor (>70 years instead of >65 years) and integration of 2 additional factors, identified in the analysis of the WEST-cohort: congestive heart failure and prior stroke. Consecutively, points were distributed as follows: age >70 years (2 points); diabetes (3 points); hypertension (1 point); coronary heart disease (1 point); distinction between stroke and TIA for baseline event (2 points for stroke); congestive heart failure (3 points) and prior stroke (3 points). The risk groups were adjusted correspondingly: risk group 1: 0–3 points; risk group 2: 4–7 points; risk group 3: 8–15 points.

Validation of the System/Studies
After validation of the SPI-I in 4 independent cohorts [Women's Estrogen for Stroke Trial (WEST) [12], n = 525; United Kingdom Transient Ischemic Attack (UK-TIA), [13] n = 2,449; Clopidogrel versus Aspirin in Patients at Risk of Ischemic Events (CAPRIE) [14], n = 6,431, and Northern Manhattan Stroke Study (NoMaSS) [15], n = 340], the WEST cohort was used to identify new prognostic variables, and these were integrated in the SPI-II. The WEST cohort was used since it was most similar to the initial cohort of SPI-I.

Application of the SPI-II in the WEST cohort showed an outcome event in 9% of group 1, 19% of group 2 and 42% of group 3, confirming a significant ($p < 0.001$) distinction between the 3 groups. SPI-II also performed well in the three other independent cohorts: in the UK-TIA cohort, the percentages for groups 1–3 were 11, 19 and 17%, respectively, the lower percentage in group 3 probably due to the small number (6 patients) in this subgroup. In the CAPRIE cohort, the distribution was 9, 17 and 26%, in the NoMaSS cohort 16, 24 and 42%. The pooled analysis for these 3 independent cohorts showed an outcome event in 10% of group 1, 19% of group 2 and 31% of group 3, which was statistically significant. A receiver operating curve (ROC) analysis was performed, showing a higher area under the curve (AUC) for SPI-II (0.63) than SPI-I (0.59), illustrating the better performance of the new tool.

The authors concluded that SPI-II is ready to use and in its performance equal to the Hankey score, but maybe easier to handle. However, some limitations such as consideration of all stroke subtypes and application to non-research cohorts might influence further results and make another revision probably necessary.

In a recent prospective cohort of TIA (n = 1,061)/stroke (n = 10,323) patients in China [16], the SPI-II showed good but not excellent results with 15% of stroke recurrence in risk group 1, 22% in risk group 2 and 24% in risk group 3. The ROC analysis for patients with TIA and recurrent stroke resulted in an AUC of 0.58 (0.54–0.63).

Life Long after Cerebral Ischemia Score (LiLAC) [17]

Background

The aim was to evaluate the very long-term outcome at 10 years after TIA or minor stroke [17] in patients with an arterial cause (patients with cardiac source of embolism were excluded). Therefore, the data of the Dutch TIA Trial (DTT) [18] were analyzed.

Definition of the System

The original publication did not have the primary goal to develop a prognostic score but Cox regression model hazard ratios (HR) for some predictive factors were calculated and therefore could be used for prospective evaluation. Considered risk factors were age, male sex, diabetes mellitus, peripheral arterial disease, index event stroke versus TIA, paresis and dysarthria. The HR were transformed into β-coefficients (= ln HR) and further processed in a complex formula [19].

Validation

2,473 participants of the DTT were investigated and followed for a mean of 10.1 years. Event-free survival after 10 years was 48%. Predictors of vascular events were the same as those in the DTT for short-time-prognosis: Age and sex-adjusted HR were 3.33 (2.97–3.73) for age over 65 years, 2.10 (1.79–2.48) for diabetes, 1.77 (1.45–2.15) for claudication, 1.94 (1.42–2.65) for previous peripheral vascular surgery, and 1.50 (1.31–1.71) for pathological Q waves on baseline electrocardiogram. After falling in the first 3 years, yearly risk of a vascular event increased over time.

Essen Stroke Risk Score (ESRS) [14, 20]

Background

In this comprehensive approach to describe risk scores after TIA, the ESRS should be mentioned quickly. Even if not developed specifically for TIA patients, it represents a tool for risk prediction of stroke and has been developed out of the CAPRIE trial [14].

Definition of the System
Based on the results of CAPRIE, a 10-point scale was developed and distribution was as follows: age 65–75 years (1 point); age >75 years (2 points); arterial hypertension (1 point); diabetes mellitus (1 point); previous MI (1 point); other cardiovascular disease (except MI and AF; 1 point); peripheral arterial disease (1 point); smoker (1 point); previous TIA or ischemic stroke in addition to qualifying event (1 point). The maximum score is 9 points, and risk groups were divided into low risk (0–2 points) and higher risk (≥3 points).

Validation
A validation was performed in a prospectively collected cohort of 852 patients with TIA or ischemic stroke in German stroke units. Patients with an ESRS score ≥3 points had a significantly higher risk of recurrent stroke (6.9 vs. 3.7%) confirming the utility of the system [20]. Validation was also performed in the European Stroke Prevention study 2 (ESPS-2).

A modified ESRS has been proposed and validated in 2012, including waist circumference, stroke subtype, and gender as additional predictive factors [21].

Comparative Studies

Prospective Comparison of ESRS, SPI, Hankey Score and LiLAC [19]
In one large comparative study with evaluation of the 4 above-mentioned predictive scores (not exclusively developed for TIA but for TIA and minor stroke) [19], 1,897 patients from 16 German neurologic departments were evaluated at 1 year after TIA/minor stroke. An ROC analysis was performed, and AUCs for prediction of recurrent stroke were as follows: ESRS 0.62 (0.57–0.67), Hankey 0.62 (0.57–0.67), LiLAC 0.64 (0.59–0.69) and SPI-II 0.65 (0.60–0.70), which means that SPI-II performed marginally better than the other 3 scores.

After description of all these scores, one should keep in mind that they were not specifically developed for TIA patients, even if they have been investigated with these scores. This becomes obvious in some of the scores differentiating between stroke and TIA concerning the distribution of points. The following chapter will focus exclusively on TIA patients and the presented scores were specially built for a TIA population.

More Recent Short-Time Approaches: California Risk Score, ABCD System and Its Developments

California Risk Score [22]

Background
Discussing the importance of treatment options and workup after TIA, the focus was now put on an earlier evaluation of the outcome after TIA. At that time, only small

studies with <200 patients had been performed with the aim to analyze the short-time prognosis after TIA, e.g. at day 90.

Definition of the System
Five prognostic factors were considered, and each was given 1 point: age ≥60 years, diabetes mellitus, unilateral weakness, speech impairment and symptom duration >10 min (maximum score 5 points). The outcome was then analyzed in view of the initial score and potential correlations.

Validation of the System
The system was validated with a cohort of 1,707 patients, collected in emergency departments of 16 hospitals of Kaiser-Permanente Northern California, followed-up for 90 days after TIA [22]. The defined outcome was stroke, but hospitalization for cardiovascular events, another TIA and death were also recorded. During the observation period, strokes occurred in 180 patients (10.5%), 91 of these had a stroke within 2 days after the TIA. For other cardiovascular events, death or TIA, an occurrence in 25% of the patients was reported within 90 days. The distribution of stroke events was as follows: in patients with 0 points 0% had a stroke, with 1 point 3% had a stroke, with 2 points 7%, 3 points 11%, 4 points 15%, and in patients with 5 points 34% suffered a stroke within 90 days after TIA. The authors did not recommend a cutoff point for high-risk/low-risk patients, and recommend validation in an independent cohort to confirm these predictive risk factors.

ABCD [6]

Background
Several approaches in the 1990s have been described above; however, they had a long-term approach rather than evaluating the risk for recurrent stroke within a short time window. Rothwell et al. [6] therefore developed a score to determine the 7-day risk (this was the suggested time frame in the North American and UK Guidelines to investigate patients with suspected TIA) of stroke after TIA and called it the ABCD score.

Definition of the System
ABCD is an acronym for Age, Blood pressure, Clinical features and Duration of symptoms. The fourth category indicates that we are dealing with a specific score for TIA patients only (and not additional minor stroke as in previous scoring systems). Points were distributed as follows: age >60 years is 1 point; blood pressure systolic >140 mm Hg or diastolic ≥90 mm Hg is 1 point; considering the clinical features, a unilateral weakness is 2 points, whereas a speech disturbance without weakness is only 1 point and other symptoms (e.g. hemihypesthesia) is 0 points. For the duration of symptoms ≥60 min of symptom duration is 2 points, 10–59 min is 1 point and <10 min is 0 points. This leads to a maximum score of 6 points.

Validation of the System

The score was derived from a population-based cohort of the Oxfordshire Community Stroke Project (OCSP) with 209 patients [6]. Five risk factors [age, clinical features, duration of symptoms, diabetes and hypertension (previous medication requiring treatment with medication or RR >140/90 mm Hg)] identified in previous studies as prognostic factors for stroke within 3 months after TIA [22, 23] were analyzed. Finally, the 4 factors with a significant association ($p < 0.1$) with stroke recurrence within 7 days were kept for the final scoring system as explained above.

The validation was performed in a cohort of the Oxford Vascular Study (OXVASC) a similar population-based study with 190 patients. The 7-day stroke risk after TIA was 10.5%. Considering the scoring system, it revealed to be highly predictive of stroke, since only 1 patient with a score <5 suffered a recurrent stroke (interestingly, this patient had diabetes, which was not part of the score), but 35.5% of the patients with a score of 6 points had a stroke within 7 days.

Finally, a pooled analysis of the OCSP and OXVASC population-based cohort (n = 377) and an analysis of a non-OXVASC hospital-referred TIA clinic (n = 206) were performed. For OXVASC, 95% of the strokes occurred in patients with a score >5; in patients with a score <5, the risk for early stroke recurrence was 0.4%, with 5 points 12.1% and with 6 points 31.4%. The corresponding ROC analysis showed a large AUC of 0.91 (0.86–0.95). In the TIA clinic analysis, no events occurred with a score <4 and corresponding results for higher scores were obtained as in the population-based cohort, albeit with less statistical power [ROC analysis with AUC 0.80 (0.72–0.89)].

In a Greek retrospective hospital-based study with 226 patients, ABCD showed a good prediction with no stroke recurrence in patients with a score of 0–2, 3.5% in patients with score 3, 7.4% score 4, 21.3% score 5 and 31.3% score 6 within 30 days after TIA, which was significant for a linear trend ($p = 0.0008$) [24]. After adjustment for stroke risk factors, history of previous TIA, medication use before the index TIA, and secondary prevention treatments, an ABCD score ≥5 was associated with an 8-fold elevated risk for recurrent stroke during the observation period ($p < 0.001$).

This score has had a large echo in the world of stroke neurologists, and has been evaluated many times in different constellations. Since most of these studies have been performed with ABCD but also further developed scores (e.g. ABCD^2 etc., see below), results will be displayed later.

ABCD^2 [25]

Background

The California Risk Score group and the ABCD group teamed up to optimize the prediction of very early stroke recurrence after TIA with the aim to obtain a scoring system which can predict the 2-day stroke risk after TIA [25]. This refined score was called the ABCD^2.

Definition of the System

Compared to the ABCD, a fifth variable, Diabetes was added (represented in the D^2 in the score). Therefore, points were distributed for age >60 years 1 point; blood pressure systolic >140 mm Hg or diastolic ≥90 mm Hg 1 point; clinical features: unilateral weakness 2 points, speech disturbance without weakness 1 point, other symptoms 0 points; duration of symptoms: ≥60 min 2 points, 10–59 min 1 point, <10 min 0 points; diabetes 1 point. This leads to a maximum score of 7 points. Risk groups were divided into low risk for $ABCD^2$ <4, moderate risk for $ABCD^2$ 4–5 and high risk for $ABCD^2$ >5.

Validation

As at that time point no larger validations in independent cohorts had been performed for the California and ABCD score, in a first step, both scores were validated in four independent groups of patients (n = 2,893) coming from different settings such as emergency departments, specialized clinics or primary care. The 2-day, 7-day and 90-day stroke risk was evaluated. As a general result, there was a good reproducibility of results between the groups with a significant trend for an increased risk of stroke with rising scores. The ABCD was slightly more powerful than the California score in ROC analysis (AUC 0.60–0.79 for California, AUC 0.62–0.81 for ABCD).

All elements of the $ABCD^2$ were independent predictors of stroke risk at the 3 time points, constituting the basis for inclusion of these parameters in the new score. Evaluation with the $ABCD^2$ in the 4 independent cohorts showed the following results: The 2-day risk of stroke was 0% for score 0–1, 1–2% for score 2, 0–3% for score 3, 2–5% for score 4, 3–7% for score 5, 4–14% for score 6 and 0–50% for score 7. With an AUC from 0.62 to 0.83, $ABCD^2$ proved to be slightly more powerful than California or ABCD (even if statistically not significant). Again, with higher scores, a higher risk for stroke was statistically confirmed and this for all 3 time points evaluated in the study. According to these results, a risk group classification was determined: $ABCD^2$ <4 was considered low risk; $ABCD^2$ 4–5 moderate risk; $ABCD^2$ >5 high risk. Considering the whole study cohort (4 independent cohorts + 2 defining cohorts; n = 4,746 patients), 130 strokes occurred within 2 days, of which 111 (85%) happened in patients not admitted to hospital. With a policy of hospital admission for moderate and high-risk patients based on the $ABCD^2$ system, only 9% of strokes (11 patients) would have occurred in patients not admitted to hospital, indicating that most of the patients with recurrent stroke would have been identified in the acute situation. Further validation of $ABCD^2$ was planned in the EXPRESS study.

The large amount of studies using the ABCD and $ABCD^2$ has been summarized in a systematic review in 2010, which had at this time identified 20 evaluated cohorts [5]. As a general observation, ABCD and $ABCD^2$ use easily assessable clinical variables. Sixteen studies used both the ABCD and $ABCD^2$ to predict stroke recurrence at 7 days, and the pooled AUC was 0.72 (0.66–0.78) for ABCD and 0.72 (0.63–0.82) for $ABCD^2$, confirming the predictive value of the scores. A significant variability of the predictive value was obvious, but mostly depended on methodological issues.

However, some studies have questioned the prognostic value of the ABCD system, underlining the potential importance of other clinical information, etiological findings and imaging findings to be integrated into the score.

In a population-based study with 284 patients, the predictive value of an $ABCD^2$ score >4 was confirmed, but 25% of the patients with recurrent stroke were missed with this scoring interpretation [26]. Addition of other clinical variables such as history of hypertension and hyperglycemia on presentation were integrated in novel scores such as AB^2CD (B^2 for history of arterial hypertension), AB^2CD^2, $ABCD^3$ (D^3 for hyperglycemia) or AB^2CD^3 and increased the sensitivity of prediction. However, even with the AB^2CD^3 system, 11% of the patients with recurrent stroke remained in the low-risk group with a score ≤4.

In a prospective study with 117 patients, ABCD scores were also analyzed in view of imaging parameters (DWI positive or negative) [27]. There, ABCD only poorly correlated with imaging parameters, many patients had a DWI lesion despite a low score. Since only 2 patients of the cohort developed stroke within 90 days (ABCD score 3 and 6), a reasonable interpretation of these data analyzing the utility of ABCD was not possible.

The results of a Spanish group analyzing 83 consecutive TIA patients from their emergency department indicated that the association of symptom duration ≥1 h and DWI abnormalities was an independent predictor of further cerebral ischemic events [28]. Besides, large artery disease (LAD), as in some previous studies, was found to be an independent predictor of recurrent stroke. However, both detected factors are not part of the ABCD, and in a following study with 345 consecutive TIA patients, this score could not predict stroke recurrence in a valuable manner (ABCD <1 risk 7.7%; 2 points 6.1%; 3 points 5.5%; 4 points 2.9%; 5 points 5.6%; 6 points 6.1%), indicating that clinical data alone might not be sufficient for a valid risk prediction [29].

A French group analyzed the predictive value of $ABCD^2$, DWI positivity and, as etiologic information, the presence of LAD and AF [30]. The outcome parameter was ischemic stroke at 1 week and 3 months after the initial TIA. For strokes within 7 days, these occurred in patients with positive DWI findings except one, stressing the importance of imaging results. Statistically, a high $ABCD^2$ score and positive DWI findings were associated with an increased risk of stroke at both end points. At 3 months, an $ABCD^2$ >5, DWI-positive imaging and LAD independently predicted an increased risk of recurrent stroke, whereas AF was not significantly associated with higher rates of stroke recurrence.

In a further study of a population-based cohort from Northern Ireland with 700 suspected TIA cases and 443 confirmed TIA cases, $ABCD^2$ had a predictive value in patients with suspected TIA evaluated by non-specialists, but for patients with diagnosis confirmed by a neurologist, the predictive value was no longer significant. Again, it was the presence of a carotid stenosis, which independently predicted the risk of stroke recurrence [31].

Several points have been brought up to explain the different performance of the same scores in different studies: the design of the studies, the methods of data collection, the clinical setting and as probably the most important point the difference in estimation of patients due to the first contact with a specialized vascular neurologist or an untrained non-neurologist in the emergency department. As illustrated in the last study, the predictive value of such scores has sometimes been attributed to the fact that non-TIAs (stroke mimics) and TIAs were distinguished and that the scores might be useful for non-specialists [32].

The ABCD and ABCD^2 are simple clinical scores which do not need complex further investigations and therefore are easily applicable in the clinical routine with collection of anamnestic details and a clinical examination. However, since these scores have not yet predicted stroke recurrence perfectly, the question was if other aspects might help to improve prediction, e.g. imaging findings (DWI positive on MRI?), knowledge about vascular status (ipsilateral stenosis?) or the stroke etiology (AF on ECG at admission?), as suggested by some studies that have been mentioned above.

The goal to further improve prediction of recurrent stroke led to several attempts to include imaging parameters in prediction scores. A systematic review in 2007 showed that the presence of acute ischemic lesions on DWI correlated with several clinical points which are part of the ABCD, and that the independent predictive value of DWI was unclear [33]. Consequently, it was only a matter of time until predictive scores including imaging results were developed.

ABCD^2 + MRI [47]

Background

After some evidence that MRI patterns might influence the prediction of stroke risk, an attempt to integrate such factors in the ABCD^2 was performed.

Definition of the System

The system is based on the ABCD^2 score, but an additional point for a DWI lesion or presence of mismatch on MRI was distributed as well as one point for evidence of intracranial vessel occlusion. This leads to the following distribution of points: age >60 years 1 point; blood pressure systolic >140 mm Hg or diastolic ≥90 mm Hg 1 point; clinical features: unilateral weakness 2 points, speech disturbance without weakness 1 point, other symptoms 0 points; duration of symptoms: ≥60 min 2 points, 10–59 min 1 point, <10 min 0 points; diabetes 1 point; presence of MRI lesions (DWI lesion and/or presence of mismatch) 1 point; evidence of intracranial vessel occlusion 1 point. This leads to a maximum score of 9 points. Risk groups were divided into low risk for 0–4, moderate risk for 5–6 and high risk for 7–9 points.

Validation

The score was derived from a study with 180 ischemic stroke patients, 87 of them had a TIA. From the univariate analyses, 8 predictive risk factors were identified, 5 being those of the ABCD^2 system and 3 additional factors assessed by MR imaging (DWI lesion status, presence of mismatch, and intracranial vessel occlusion). In this cohort, $ABCD^2$ + MRI predicted stroke recurrence significantly better than the simple $ABCD^2$ (AUC for $ABCD^2$ + MRI 0.88; $ABCD^2$ 0.78). The arbitrary risk group definition showed that patients with a presumed high risk (7–9 points) had 32.1%, the intermediate group (5–6 points) 5.4%, and the low risk group (0–4 points) 0% of stroke recurrence.

Clinical- and Imaging-Based Prediction of Stroke Risk after Transient Ischemic Attack: The CIP Model [34]

Background

With the aim to optimize stroke prediction within 7 days after TIA, the authors hypothesized that imaging criteria might independently predict stroke recurrence and therefore that a combination of $ABCD^2$ and DWI positivity would improve prediction [34]. This prediction model based on clinical and imaging criteria was thus called the CIP model.

Definition of the System

The approach consists in the application of the $ABCD^2$ score, dichotomization of the score into $ABCD^2$ ≤4 and >4 and consideration if a patient was DWI positive or negative on MRI. Subsequently, patients with $ABCD^2$ >4 and DWI positive on MRI or positive on MRI alone are considered at high risk.

Validation

In a retrospective analysis of 601 consecutive patients with TIA who underwent DWI-MRI within 24 h after symptoms, $ABCD^2$ and DWI-positive MRI were independent predictors of stroke risk. The 7-day risk for stroke was 2.0% with an $ABCD^2$ score ≥4 alone, 4.9% with acute infarct on diffusion-weighted imaging alone, and 14.9% with a combination of $ABCD^2$ ≥4 and DWI-positive MRI. In other words, the power of the analysis improved with addition of DWI to the $ABCD^2$, since the AUC of the ROC analysis was 0.66 (0.57–0.76) for $ABCD^2$ alone, 0.76 (0.67–0.86) for DWI MRI alone and 0.79 (0.72–0.86) after correction for the combined score. An automated calculator on the Internet is available (http://cip.martinos.org) to calculate the risk constellation immediately.

$ABCD^2I$ [35]

Background

As already stated in some publications after development of the ABCD score, imaging parameters such as DWI-positive MRI have been claimed to improve risk prediction for stroke after TIA. Therefore, the creators of ABCD initiated an international, multicenter collaborative study to determine the prognostic performance of the $ABCD^2$ with additional brain infarction on imaging. This system was then called the $ABCD^2I$.

Definition of the System

The system is based on the $ABCD^2$. Additionally, imaging criteria were included. This led to the following distribution of points: age >60 years 1 point; blood pressure systolic >140 mm Hg or diastolic ≥90 mm Hg 1 point; clinical features: unilateral weakness 2 points, speech disturbance without weakness 1 point, other symptoms 0 points; duration of symptoms: ≥60 min 2 points, 10–59 min 1 point, <10 min 0 points; diabetes 1 point and brain infarction on imaging [either DWI (any acute infarction) or CT (any infarction irrespective of presenting symptoms)] 3 points. The maximum score is 10 points. Specific risk groups were not defined.

Validation

In the multicenter study with 4,574 patients, 27.6% had acute infarction on DWI (performed in 3,206 patients) and 23.9% had infarction on CT (performed in 1,368 patients) [35] confirming the presence of acute infarction in about 1/3 of TIA patients in previous studies. Brain infarction on imaging was defined as 'any acute infarction, irrespective of whether it was appropriate to the presenting symptoms' on DWI, and 'any infarction (given the unreliability of distinction between acute and old infarction)' on CT. There was a slight tendency towards infarction on DWI being a more powerful predictor of stroke than infarction on CT. The discriminatory power for stroke within 7 and 90 days after TIA as measured by the AUC was evaluated for $ABCD^2$ and for $ABCD^2I$ with 3 different weightings of imaging criteria (1–3 points). The greatest improvement in the predictive power of $ABCD^2I$ was observed when the infarction component was weighted with 3 points [AUC for $ABCD^2$ 0.66 (0.53–0.78), for $ABCD^2I$ with 3 points 0.78 (0.72 to 0.85)]. Besides the results for the pooled analysis of all 12 cohorts, individual analyses of each cohort (except for 2) also showed a better predictive power of the new $ABCD^2I$ score than $ABCD^2$ alone.

$ABCD^3$ and $ABCD^3I$ [36]

Background

With the $ABCD^2I$, evidence has been provided that addition of imaging parameters improves the risk prediction for stroke after TIA. Other factors, such as carotid stenosis have also been associated with an elevated risk of stroke after TIA. The aim was now to improve (a) the $ABCD^2$ as a score for the preclinical situation (the $ABCD^3$ score) and (b) to evaluate if an optimized score for secondary care could be found (the $ABCD^3I$ score).

Definition of the Systems

ABCD^3

This score was based again on the ABCD^2 with additional assessment of a history of prior TIA within 1 week before the index event. The score therefore was composed by these factors: age >60 years 1 point; blood pressure systolic >140 mm Hg or diastolic ≥90 mm Hg 1 point; clinical features: unilateral weakness 2 points, speech disturbance without weakness 1 point, other symptoms 0 points; duration of symptoms: ≥60 min 2 points, 10–59 min 1 point, <10 min 0 points; diabetes 1 point and prior TIA within 1 week 2 points, making a maximum of 9 points. Risk groups were divided into low risk (0–3 points), intermediate risk (4–5 points) and high risk (6–9 points).

ABCD^{3}I

Based on the ABCD^3, the ABCD^{3}I integrated information on vascular investigations and imaging results, which resulted in the following score constellation: age >60 years 1 point; blood pressure systolic >140 mm Hg or diastolic ≥90 mm Hg 1 point; clinical features: unilateral weakness 2 points, speech disturbance without weakness 1 point, other symptoms 0 points; duration of symptoms: ≥60 min 2 points, 10–59 min 1 point, <10 min 0 points; diabetes 1 point and prior TIA within 1 week 2 points, stenosis on carotid imaging (>50%) 2 points and abnormal DWI 2 points, making a maximum of 13 points. Risk groups were divided into low risk (0–3 points), intermediate risk (4–7 points) and high risk (8–13 points).

Validation

The derivation sample for development of the improved scores contained 2,654 patients [36]. The results generated with these data were validated in another cohort of 1,232 patients.

In a first step, the ABCD^3 score was analyzed with regard to the preexisting ABCD^2. In the derivation sample, ABCD^3 showed better results than ABCD^2, but in the validation sample results were of similar predictive value. The authors therefore concluded that more studies were needed to evaluate if ABCD^3 really performs better and should replace ABCD^2 in daily routine.

In a second step, ABCD^{3}I results were analyzed and the categorization in low, medium and high-risk showed a significant trend for increasing stroke recurrence at 2, 7, 28 and 90 days with higher risk scores. ABCD^{3}I showed a better discrimination of patients at high risk for early stroke recurrence [AUC at day 7 in the validation sample 0.71 (0.63–0.78) for ABCD^{3}I, 0.63 (0.56–0.69) for ABCD^2, similar significant tendencies for day 28 and day 90]. Therefore, one could conclude that ABCD^{3}I provides an improvement of risk stratification in secondary care settings.

In a Chinese study, which analyzed stroke recurrence at days 2 and 7, ABCD^{3}I also proved to be highly effective for prediction of recurrent stroke in a sample of 107 patients (AUC at day 2 for ABCD^2, ABCD^3 and ABCD^{3}I were 0.61, 0.66 and 0.71) [37].

Since recently the definition of TIA has been discussed, and the importance of imaging findings in risk prediction for recurrent stroke has been shown in several studies, one should cite a large study with 4,574 TIA patients from 12 European stroke centers [38]. Patients with a DWI lesion (n = 3,206) had a significantly higher recurrence of stroke in the first 7 days (7.1%) than DWI-negative patients (0.4%). The $ABCD^2$ score, however, had a predictive value in both cohorts [DWI-positive patients: AUC 0.68 (0.63–0.73), DWI-negative patients: AUC 0.73 (0.67–0.80)]. Since DWI-positive patients with a low $ABCD^2$ score had a similar stroke risk as DWI-negative patients with high $ABCD^2$, the authors concluded, that imaging results should always be considered. This might also be a CT scan in cases where MRI is not available, as supported by their data as well.

ASPIRE Approach [39]

Background

With the aim to always better stratify the risk for recurrent stroke, many groups tried to optimize the tools for stroke prediction. Since the imaging criteria are not always available and the scoring system was initially created as a simple clinical score, some investigators tried to develop guidelines based on easily available information but going beyond the classical $ABCD^2$ approach.

Definition of the System

The approach in the Alberta province in Canada consisted in calculating the $ABCD^2$ and then considering additional information [39]. Patients with $ABCD^2$ score ≥4, or motor or speech symptoms lasting >5 min, or with AF were considered as high-risk patients. This was called the ASPIRE approach.

Validation

This approach was tested retrospectively analyzing the 90-day stroke risk of 573 consecutive patients diagnosed with TIA. It had a 100% negative predictive value since with this classification no low-risk patient suffered a stroke. This was an advantage compared to $ABCD^2$, where 2 patients with a score <4 suffered recurrent strokes. In the ASPIRE high-risk group, 6.3% of patients had a stroke during follow-up. However, with this new system a large majority (78% of the study population) were classified as high-risk patients, which is against the idea to make a meaningful triage of TIA patients in the acute situation.

ABCDE+ [40]

Background

Obviously, the ongoing development of scoring systems to predict stroke recurrence after TIA reflects the relevance of the topic, and despite all efforts the need for further improvement. Regardless of a low score in $ABCD^2$, some patients suffer from recurrent stroke after TIA. Previous scores had taken into account a carotid stenosis ($ABCD^3I$) or AF (ASPIRE approach), reflecting the potential predictive value of the determined etiology. Therefore one of the last approaches has been to develop a new score on the basis of $ABCD^2$, which additionally includes the etiology as well as findings on DWI.

Definition of the System

The basis of this score was $ABCD^2$. Additionally etiologic findings were integrated with different weighting factors according to the etiology; DWI positivity was also considered as a predictive factor [40]. Therefore, the scoring was as follows: age >60 years 1 point; blood pressure systolic >140 mm Hg or diastolic ≥90 mm Hg 1 point; clinical features: unilateral weakness 2 points, speech disturbance without weakness 1 point, other symptoms 0 points; duration of symptoms: ≥60 min 2 points, 10–59 min 1 point, <10 min 0 points; diabetes 1 point; etiology: LAD 3 points; cardioembolism 1 point; undetermined 1 point; small vessel disease 0 points; other 0 points; DWI positive 3 points. The score was named ABCDE+ ('E' for etiology and '+' for additional imaging parameters). The level of risk was arbitrarily set as high risk for >6 points and as low risk for ≤6.

Validation of the System

The score was created based on a prospective cohort study of 248 consecutive TIA patients in emergency departments of a university hospital in Switzerland. The outcome at 90 days after TIA was evaluated. Patients who fulfilled the following 4 criteria were treated as outpatients (and therefore considered as low risk): an ABCD score ≤4, no DWI lesion, <50% stenosis of large arteries and absence of high-risk abnormality on ECG. All other patients were hospitalized.

With the risk stratification with ABCDE+ (high risk >6) compared to ABCD (high risk >4), 29.8% of patients were reclassified. Out of the 28 patients (more than the half of them had stroke recurrence within the first 7 days), who suffered recurrent stroke, 12 were shifted from the low to the high-risk group with ABCDE+. Only one patient with recurrent stroke was reclassified from high to low risk. Consequently, ROC analysis showed better performance with an AUC of 0.67 (0.55–0.75) for ABCDE+ compared to 0.50 (0.40–0.61) for ABCD and 0.48 (0.37–0.58) for $ABCD^2$ ($p = 0.04$). The difference between ABCDE+ and $ABCD^2$ was significant ($p = 0.04$); between ABCDE+ and ABCD, there was a tendency ($p = 0.07$).

Since this was the validation cohort, further trials in independent cohorts are needed. One should also address the problem of what to do with patients who did not undergo MRI with DWI since they cannot be classified with the ABCDE+. The alternative possibility (as done in the $ABCD^3I$ study) to use CT information was not assessed in the study.

Comparative Studies for Validation of Different Scores

PROMAPA Study [41]
In the PROMAPA study, several scores for prediction of recurrent stroke such as the ABCD, $ABCD^2$, $ABCD^2I$, $ABCD^3$, California Risk Score, ESRS and SPI-II were analyzed in a prospectively collected cohort of 1,137 patients from 30 Spanish stroke centers [41]. The 7-day risk of stroke and 90-day risk of stroke were determined. The predictive value of $ABCD^3$ was confirmed at 7 days [AUC 0.66 (0.54–0.77)] and 90 days [AUC 0.61 (0.52–0.70)]. In the study, a new $ABCD^3V$ score with 2 additional points for ≥50% of symptomatic stenosis on carotid or intracranial imaging was created, improving the results of the basically used $ABCD^3$ [7- and 90-day outcome: AUC 0.69 (0.57–0.81) and AUC 0.63 (0.51–0.69), respectively, with $ABCD^3V$]. Furthermore, prior TIA and LAD were confirmed as independent predictors of stroke recurrence. As a consequence, all scores that do not take into account vascular imaging or prior TIA failed to predict stroke recurrence in TIA patients in statistical analysis. These results contradict the findings of several pre-existing studies and the review about some of these scales. One explanation might be the lower rate of stroke recurrence in the PROMAPA study, therefore not permitting to generate significant results with the applied scores. Another distractor might be the setting with an evaluation by stroke neurologists rather than non-specialists in the primary clinical setting. However, this study demonstrates that the simple scoring systems exclusively based on clinical information might fail to predict the risk for stroke recurrence and therefore cannot be used as the only decision tool when deciding whether to keep a patient at hospital or send him to an outpatient setting.

Prediction of a First Transient Ischemic Attack/Stroke

Stroke Risk Stratification in Atrial Fibrillation

This topic represents another very important aspect of risk for TIA, which could itself fill a whole chapter or book. Since risk stratification scores in AF have not been specifically developed to evaluate TIA patients, we will only provide an additional but short overview. One parallel to the risk prediction after TIA is a large variety of scores and approaches. Like the ABCD system, the $CHADS^2$ system and its refinements are the most widely applied score in clinical routine and therefore are presented in this chapter.

Overview on Existing Scores [42]
In 2008, a comprehensive overview of 12 schemes developed for prediction of stroke in AF was published [42]. Seven scores were based on event-rate analyses, the other 5 scores were derived from expert consensus meetings. Four schemes integrated clinical information only; in 7 approaches results from echocardiography were considered.

The most frequently included features were previous stroke/TIA (100% of the scores), age (83%), hypertension (83%), and diabetes (83%). However, despite some similarities, evaluation of the scores showed important discrepancies in risk prediction and therefore further refinement of scores was suggested.

CHADS2 [48]
CHADS is an acronym for Cardiac failure, Hypertension, Age, Diabetes and Stroke. For each factor, 1 point is distributed, except for the history of stroke, which is given 2 points (therefore the '2' in the score). In a study of 1,733 patients with non-valvular AF, the risk of stroke during follow-up was analyzed with 3 evaluation schemes, which were the system of the Atrial Fibrillation Investigators (AFI), the Stroke Prevention in Atrial Fibrillation (SPAF) III and the new CHADS2. The results of CHADS2 were promising with a stroke rate per 100 patient-years (without antithrombotic therapy) increasing by a factor of 1.5 for each 1-point increase: 1.9 for score 0; 2.8 for 1; 4.0 for 2; 5.9 for 3; 8.5 for 4; 12.5 for 5, and 18.2 for 6. The actual interpretation is a low risk for patients with 0 points, moderate risk for 1 point and a high risk for 2–6 points.

CHA2DS2-VASc [43]
Further refinement of the CHADS2 was needed, and therefore CHA2DS2-VASc was developed. It stands for cardiac failure of dysfunction, hypertension, age ≥75 years diabetes, stroke, vascular disease, age 65–74, sex category (female) [43]. The score was validated in a cohort of 1,084 patients and showed an increased occurrence of thromboembolic events with higher scores. 'Major (definitive)' risk factors were defined as previous stroke/TIA, age ≥75 years. 'Clinically relevant non-major' risk factors are: heart failure, hypertension, diabetes, female gender, age 65–74 years, and atherosclerotic vascular disease. With 1 major risk factor or a CHA2DS2-VASc score ≥1, indication for anticoagulation is given following cardiologic guideline recommendations.

Epidemiological Studies and Scores

Epidemiological studies on the risk to develop stroke have not been specifically designed to predict occurrence of a first TIA. However, since TIA represents a subdivision of clinical stroke subtype, a short overview of studies predicting the risk for a first stroke (based on a risk score) is provided in this chapter.

The Framingham Study [44]

From the results of the Framingham study cohort, a mathematical function has been developed for the prediction of stroke [44]. Predictive stroke risk factors included age (0–10 points according to the age between 54–86 years), systolic blood pressure (0–10 points according to values between 95–213 mm Hg), use of antihypertensive therapy (2 points), diabetes mellitus (2 points), cigarette smoking (3 points), prior cardiovascular disease (coronary heart disease, cardiac failure, or intermittent claudication; 3 points), AF (4 points), and left ventricular hypertrophy by ECG (6 points). 472 strokes occurred during 10 years' follow-up with a significant growing probability correlated with the number of points in the score.

In a further attempt to optimize the score and to include effects of treatment interventions during the study, an adjustment for antihypertensive medication has been made [45].

The EUROSTROKE Study [46]

In a large epidemiological approach of 10 European research centers evaluating the risk of stroke in men in the general population (aged 40–85 years), significant independent predictive risk factors were identified: increasing age, a history of stroke, diabetes, current smoking, a history of hypertension and an elevated diastolic blood pressure [46]. A model was built based on the odds ratios and regression coefficients of these factors, calculating a final score predictive of the stroke risk of each individual. Composition of the score was: age (per year) 0.3; history of stroke 19; diabetes 8; current smoking 5; history of hypertension 3; diastolic blood pressure (mm Hg) 0.2. Stroke occurred in 1.0% of subjects with a score <30, 1.4% with a score 30–35, 2.4% with a score 36–40, 5.2% with a score 41–45, 4.5% with a score 46–50 and 14.2% with a score >50. Therefore, the authors of the study decided to put an arbitrary threshold at 41 points, distinguishing between low- and high-risk subjects. The ROC analysis of this model resulted in an AUC of 0.69; the sensitivity to predict all future stroke cases was 40% with a specificity of 85%. The addition of other potential predictive factors such as pulse rate, body mass index, blood lipids, fibrinogen level and ECG parameters did not improve the classification of subjects.

Conclusions

Development of scores to stratify the risk for recurrent stroke after TIA has been of interest since the 1990s. In a first attempt, the focus was put on the long-term outcome, reflected by systems such as the SPI and Hankey score. In the 2000s, clinical decision-making became rather important, and scores have been developed for application in emergency department situations to distinguish between patients with high- and low-risk for stroke recurrence in the early course (2–7 days after TIA). The most prominent score is the ABCD system. With the aim to always improve and optimize the risk stratification, several approaches and investigations have been performed. The best and currently recommended score for primary clinical use is the $ABCD^2$. However, with technical investigation being more and more available through the years, factors such as DWI findings or etiologic results (detection of carotid stenosis or AF) were integrated into these systems in the 2010s, e.g. the ABCD^{3}I. These new scores have a high predictive value but represent scores for secondary care in large stroke centers rather than for primary care in the emergency department. Therefore, before applying a score to evaluate the patient, the physician should always keep his clinical judgment in mind and never neglect the individual examination of the patient.

References

1 Giles MF, Rothwell PM: Risk of stroke early after transient ischaemic attack: a systematic review and meta-analysis. Lancet Neurol 2007;6:1063–1072.

2 Rothwell PM, Warlow CP: Timing of TIAs preceding stroke: time window for prevention is very short. Neurology 2005;64:817–820.

3 Brainin M, McShane LM, Steiner M, Dachenhausen A, Seiser A: Silent brain infarcts and transient ischemic attacks. A three-year study of first-ever ischemic stroke patients: the Klosterneuburg Stroke Data Bank. Stroke 1995;26:1348–1352.

4 D'Agostino RB Sr, Grundy S, Sullivan LM, Wilson P: Validation of the Framingham coronary heart disease prediction scores: results of a multiple ethnic groups investigation. JAMA 2001;286:180–187.

5 Giles MF, Rothwell PM: Systematic review and pooled analysis of published and unpublished validations of the ABCD and ABCD2 transient ischemic attack risk scores. Stroke 2010;41:667–673.

6 Rothwell PM, Giles MF, Flossmann E, Lovelock CE, Redgrave JN, Warlow CP, et al: A simple score (ABCD) to identify individuals at high early risk of stroke after transient ischaemic attack. Lancet 2005;366:29–36.

7 Kernan WN, Horwitz RI, Brass LM, Viscoli CM, Taylor KJ: A prognostic system for transient ischemia or minor stroke. Ann Intern Med 1991;114:552–557.

8 A randomized trial of aspirin and sulfinpyrazone in threatened stroke. The Canadian Cooperative Study Group. N Engl J Med 1978;299:53–59.

9 Kernan WN, Viscoli CM, Brass LM, Makuch RW, Sarrel PM, Roberts RS, et al: The stroke prognosis instrument II (SPI-II): A clinical prediction instrument for patients with transient ischemia and nondisabling ischemic stroke. Stroke 2000;31:456–462.

10 Hankey GJ, Slattery JM, Warlow CP: Transient ischaemic attacks: which patients are at high (and low) risk of serious vascular events? J Neurol Neurosurg Psychiatry 1992;55:640–652.

11 Hankey GJ, Slattery JM, Warlow CP: Can the long term outcome of individual patients with transient ischaemic attacks be predicted accurately? J Neurol Neurosurg Psychiatry 1993;56:752–759.

12 Kernan WN, Brass LM, Viscoli CM, Sarrel PM, Makuch R, Horwitz RI: Estrogen after ischemic stroke: clinical basis and design of the Women's Estrogen for Stroke Trial. J Stroke Cerebrovasc Dis 1998;7:85–95.

13 Farrell B, Godwin J, Richards S, Warlow C: The United Kingdom transient ischaemic attack (UK-TIA) aspirin trial: final results. J Neurol Neurosurg Psychiatry 1991;54:1044–1054.

14 CAPRIE Steering Committee: A randomised, blinded, trial of clopidogrel versus aspirin in patients at risk of ischaemic events (CAPRIE). CAPRIE Steering Committee. Lancet 1996;348:1329–1339.

15 Sacco RL, Kargman DE, Gu Q, Zamanillo MC: Race-ethnicity and determinants of intracranial atherosclerotic cerebral infarction. The Northern Manhattan Stroke Study. Stroke 1995;26:14–20.

16 Meng X, Wang Y, Zhao X, Wang C, Li H, Liu L, et al: Validation of the Essen Stroke Risk Score and the Stroke Prognosis Instrument II in Chinese patients. Stroke 2011;42:3619–3620.

17 van Wijk I, Kappelle LJ, van Gijn J, Koudstaal PJ, Franke CL, Vermeulen M, et al: Long-term survival and vascular event risk after transient ischaemic attack or minor ischaemic stroke: a cohort study. Lancet 2005;365:2098–2104.

18 A comparison of two doses of aspirin (30 vs. 283 mg a day) in patients after a transient ischemic attack or minor ischemic stroke. The Dutch TIA Trial Study Group. N Engl J Med 1991;325:1261–1266.

19 Weimar C, Benemann J, Michalski D, Muller M, Luckner K, Katsarava Z, et al: Prediction of recurrent stroke and vascular death in patients with transient ischemic attack or nondisabling stroke: a prospective comparison of validated prognostic scores. Stroke 2010;41:487–493.

20 Weimar C, Goertler M, Rother J, Ringelstein EB, Darius H, Nabavi DG, et al: Predictive value of the Essen Stroke Risk Score and Ankle Brachial Index in acute ischaemic stroke patients from 85 German stroke units. J Neurol Neurosurg Psychiatry 2008;79: 1339–1343.
21 Sumi S, Origasa H, Houkin K, Terayama Y, Uchiyama S, Daida H, et al: A modified Essen stroke risk score for predicting recurrent cardiovascular events: development and validation. Int J Stroke 2013;8: 251–257.
22 Johnston SC, Gress DR, Browner WS, Sidney S: Short-term prognosis after emergency department diagnosis of TIA. JAMA 2000;284:2901–2906.
23 Hill MD, Yiannakoulias N, Jeerakathil T, Tu JV, Svenson LW, Schopflocher DP: The high risk of stroke immediately after transient ischemic attack: a population-based study. Neurology 2004;62:2015–2020.
24 Tsivgoulis G, Spengos K, Manta P, Karandreas N, Zambelis T, Zakopoulos N, et al: Validation of the ABCD score in identifying individuals at high early risk of stroke after a transient ischemic attack: a hospital-based case series study. Stroke 2006;37:2892–2897.
25 Johnston SC, Rothwell PM, Nguyen-Huynh MN, Giles MF, Elkins JS, Bernstein AL, et al: Validation and refinement of scores to predict very early stroke risk after transient ischaemic attack. Lancet 2007; 369:283–292.
26 Fothergill A, Christianson TJ, Brown RD Jr, Rabinstein AA: Validation and refinement of the ABCD2 score: a population-based analysis. Stroke 2009;40: 2669–2673.
27 Cucchiara BL, Messe SR, Taylor RA, Pacelli J, Maus D, Shah Q, et al: Is the ABCD score useful for risk stratification of patients with acute transient ischemic attack? Stroke 2006;37:1710–1714.
28 Purroy F, Montaner J, Rovira A, Delgado P, Quintana M, Alvarez-Sabin J: Higher risk of further vascular events among transient ischemic attack patients with diffusion-weighted imaging acute ischemic lesions. Stroke 2004;35:2313–2319.
29 Purroy F, Molina CA, Montaner J, Alvarez-Sabin J: Absence of usefulness of ABCD score in the early risk of stroke of transient ischemic attack patients (letter). Stroke 2007;38:855–856, author reply 7.
30 Calvet D, Touze E, Oppenheim C, Turc G, Meder JF, Mas JL: DWI lesions and TIA etiology improve the prediction of stroke after TIA. Stroke 2009;40:187–192.
31 Sheehan OC, Kyne L, Kelly LA, Hannon N, Marnane M, Merwick A, et al: Population-based study of ABCD2 score, carotid stenosis, and atrial fibrillation for early stroke prediction after transient ischemic attack: the North Dublin TIA study. Stroke 2010;41: 844–850.
32 Josephson SA, Sidney S, Pham TN, Bernstein AL, Johnston SC: Higher ABCD2 score predicts patients most likely to have true transient ischemic attack. Stroke 2008;39:3096–3098.
33 Redgrave JN, Coutts SB, Schulz UG, Briley D, Rothwell PM: Systematic review of associations between the presence of acute ischemic lesions on diffusion-weighted imaging and clinical predictors of early stroke risk after transient ischemic attack. Stroke 2007;38:1482–1488.
34 Ay H, Arsava EM, Johnston SC, Vangel M, Schwamm LH, Furie KL, et al: Clinical- and imaging-based prediction of stroke risk after transient ischemic attack: the CIP model. Stroke 2009;40:181–186.
35 Giles MF, Albers GW, Amarenco P, Arsava MM, Asimos A, Ay H, et al: Addition of brain infarction to the ABCD2 Score (ABCD2I): a collaborative analysis of unpublished data on 4574 patients. Stroke 2010;41:1907–1913.
36 Merwick A, Albers GW, Amarenco P, Arsava EM, Ay H, Calvet D, et al: Addition of brain and carotid imaging to the ABCD(2) score to identify patients at early risk of stroke after transient ischaemic attack: a multicentre observational study. Lancet Neurol 2010;9:1060–1069.
37 Song XK, Wang WJ, Li HY, Ren MS, Wu L, Ma JF: The value of ABCD3-I score in prediction of cerebral infarction after transient ischaemic attack (in Chinese). Zhonghua Nei Ke Za Zhi 2012;51:445–448.
38 Giles MF, Albers GW, Amarenco P, Arsava EM, Asimos AW, Ay H, et al: Early stroke risk and ABCD2 score performance in tissue- vs time-defined TIA: a multicenter study. Neurology 2011;77:1222–1228.
39 Coutts SB, Sylaja PN, Choi YB, Al-Khathami A, Sivakumar C, Jeerakathil TJ, et al: The ASPIRE approach for TIA risk stratification. Can J Neurol Sci 2011;38:78–81.
40 Engelter ST, Amort M, Jax F, Weisskopf F, Katan M, Burow A, et al: Optimizing the risk estimation after a transient ischaemic attack – the ABCDE plus sign in circle score. Eur J Neurol 2012;19:55–61.
41 Purroy F, Jimenez Caballero PE, Gorospe A, Torres MJ, Alvarez-Sabin J, Santamarina E, et al: Prediction of early stroke recurrence in transient ischemic attack patients from the PROMAPA study: a comparison of prognostic risk scores. Cerebrovasc Dis 2012; 33:182–189.
42 Comparison of 12 risk stratification schemes to predict stroke in patients with nonvalvular atrial fibrillation. Stroke 2008;39:1901–1910.
43 Lip GY, Nieuwlaat R, Pisters R, Lane DA, Crijns HJ: Refining clinical risk stratification for predicting stroke and thromboembolism in atrial fibrillation using a novel risk factor-based approach: the Euro Heart Survey on atrial fibrillation. Chest 2010;137: 263–272.

44 Wolf PA, D'Agostino RB, Belanger AJ, Kannel WB: Probability of stroke: a risk profile from the Framingham Study. Stroke 1991;22:312–318.
45 D'Agostino RB, Wolf PA, Belanger AJ, Kannel WB: Stroke risk profile: adjustment for antihypertensive medication. The Framingham Study. Stroke 1994; 25:40–43.
46 Moons KG, Bots ML, Salonen JT, Elwood PC, Freire de Concalves A, Nikitin Y, et al: Prediction of stroke in the general population in Europe (EUROSTROKE): is there a role for fibrinogen and electrocardiography? J Epidemiol Community Health 2002;56(suppl 1): i30–i36.
47 Coutts SB, Eliasziw M, Hill MD, Scott JN, Subramaniam S, Buchan AM, Demchuk AM, VISION study group: An improved scoring system for identifying patients at high early risk of stroke and functional impairment after an acute transient ischemic attack or minor stroke. Int J Stroke 2008;3:3–10.
48 Gage BF, Waterman AD, Shannon W, Boechler M, Rich MW, Radford MJ: Validation of clinical classification schemes for predicting stroke: results from the National Registry of Atrial Fibrillation. JAMA 2001;285:2864–2870.

Dr. Marc E. Wolf
Department of Neurology, UniversitätsMedizin Mannheim UMM
University of Heidelberg, Theodor-Kutzer-Ufer 1–3
DE–68167 Mannheim (Germany)
E-Mail wolf@neuro.ma.uni-heidelberg.de

Uchiyama S, Amarenco P, Minematsu K, Wong KSL (eds): TIA as Acute Cerebrovascular Syndrome.
Front Neurol Neurosci. Basel, Karger, 2014, vol 33, pp 69–81 (DOI: 10.1159/000351892)

Epidemiology of Transient Ischemic Attack

Yoshihiro Kokubo

Department of Preventive Cardiology, National Cerebral and Cardiovascular Disease, Osaka, Japan

Abstract

Few epidemiologic data are available regarding the prevalence and incidence of transient ischemic attack (TIA). Here, the incidence of TIA and that of subsequent stroke events were reviewed. The incidences of TIA in Europe were 0.52–2.37 and 0.05–1.14 in men and women aged 55–64, 0.94–3.39 and 0.71–1.47 in those aged 65–74, and 3.04–7.20 and 2.18–6.06 in those aged 75–84, respectively. The corresponding incidences are similar in the United States, and lower in Japan. Higher incidences were revealed in men compared with women. The incidence of TIA increased very markedly with age, regardless of race or gender. The evidence of risk factors for TIA excluding ischemic strokes is very limited. The ABCD/ABCD^2 score was developed to predict individual risk and to triage patients on the first presentation. In prognostic TIA, the crude rate of stroke risks (%) for general populations were 1.7, 4.8, 6.6, 8.5, and 11.4 at 2 days, 1 week, 1 month, 3 and 6 months, whereas those for hospital patients were 13.7 and 12.4 at 1 and 3 months, respectively. There is very limited evidence of an association between a family history of stroke and the incidence of stroke after TIA, which showed that family history of stroke does not predict the risk of ischemic stroke after TIA. There is also limited evidence of seasonal variation in TIA incidence. TIAs were reported to be most frequent in autumn or spring and less common in winter or spring to summer, and most frequent on Mondays. There seems to be no consensus regarding seasonal differences in TIA incidence.

Transient ischemic attack (TIA) is an acute episode of temporary neurologic impairment lasting <24 h, caused by focal ischemia in the brain or retina. TIAs are variable in duration, commonly lasting from 5 to 60 min, but they occasionally last as long as 24 h, but may leave no persistent neurological deficit [1]. According

Table 1. Prevalence of TIA according to age, sex, and race/ethnic group

Population	Age, years	TIA, %		Year and reference
		men	women	
African-Americans				
Jackson, Miss., US				1996 [2]
	45–54	1.5	3.2	
	55–64	1.7	3.2	
	Total	1.6	3.2	
Forsyth, N.C., US				1996 [1]
	45–54	4.0	7.6	
	55–64	4.6	7.8	
	Total	4.3	7.7	
Evans, Ga., US				1973 [3]
	45–54	12.1	0.0	
	55–64	8.9	13.8	
	65	12.1	8.6	
European-Americans				
Forsyth, N.C., US				1996 [2]
	45–54	3.2	5.1	
	55–64	2.5	6.4	
	Total	2.9	5.7	
Evans, G.A., US				1973 [3]
	45–54	20.8	4.9	
	55–64	15.5	10.4	
	65	30.3	18.2	

to the recent American Heart Association/American Stroke Association diagnostic recommendations, TIA patients should undergo a neuroimaging evaluation within 24 h of symptom onset. Patients who have experienced a TIA are at high risk of stroke. However, there are few epidemiologic data on TIA, especially reviews of the incidence and prognostic value of TIAs. In this review, I will focus on the incidence of TIA and subsequent stroke events from an epidemiological point of view.

Prevalence and Incidence of Transient Ischemic Attack

The prevalence of TIA according to age, sex, and race/ethnic group is shown in table 1 [2, 3]. Among African-Americans, the prevalence of TIA does not seem to increase according to age in both men and women. According to the Atherosclerosis Risk in Communities (ARIC) Study, the prevalence of TIA in African-American men and women per 1,000 persons was 1.5–1.7 and around 3.2 in Jackson, Miss., but 4.0–4.6 and 7.6–7.8 in Forsyth, N.C., respectively [2]. However, in Evans County, Ga., the prevalence of TIA in the age groups 45–54, 55–64, and 65+ years was 12.1, 8.9, and 12.1 in men and 0, 13.8, and 8.6 in women per 1,000 persons, respectively [3]. These prevalence results are much higher than those obtained in Jackson and Forsyth. The data for Jackson and Forsyth are from 1996, which is 23 years after the Evans data. These two sets of data may not be compared simply because of a different generation.

In the ARIC study, the diagnosis of TIA was categorized as *definite* for a sudden onset of transient limb paralysis, with or without other signs, lasting up to 24 h and leaving no significant deficit; *probable* for other transient focal neurologic deficits lasting up to 24 h; *possible* for a less clear-cut history of symptoms or non-focal symptoms, or *vague* for anxiety and/or emotional symptoms. Evans County, is located in 'the Stroke Belt' in the south-eastern United States, which shows relatively higher stroke incidence. Therefore the prevalence of TIA in Evans County seems to be greater than in other areas.

In a European-American population in Forsyth, the prevalence of TIA was 2.9 and 5.7 in men and women per 1,000 persons, respectively. In Evans, the TIA prevalence of a European-American population was 20.8, 15.5, and 30.3 in men and 4.9, 10.4, and 18.2 in women per 1,000 persons according to the 45–54, 55–64, and 65 or older (65+) age groups, respectively. The prevalence of TIA tends to increase according to age in both men and women.

The Hisayama study examined the prevalence of TIA in the Japanese population [4]. The prevalence of TIA in the Hisayama study was 4.9 per 1,000 persons [4], less than half that in the European-American population in Evans. (13.8 per 1,000 persons) [3]. The etiology of incident TIA in Japan may be different from that in Western countries. Among the Hisayama participants with TIA, 11 subsequent cerebral infarctions were observed; they were diagnosed as 6 lacunar infarctions, 3 embolisms, and 2 atherothromboses by clinical and/or pathological finding or autopsy. The ARIC study showed that TIA due to atherosclerosis was attributable to myocardial infarction in 57% and to stroke in 38% of mortality patients (n = 37) [2]. TIAs due to atherosclerosis (which is usually of carotid artery origin) are estimated to be less common in Japan than in Western countries, and lacunar stroke might be important as an etiology of TIA in Japan [2].

As illustrated in figure 1 [4–11] and table 2, [4, 5, 7, 8, 10, 12–15] the Hisayama study found that the average incidence of the first TIA was 0.78 and 0.38 per 1,000 person-years in men and women, respectively [4]. According to community studies in the US, the average incidence rate for the first TIA was 0.31 per 1,000 person-years (0.93 per 1,000 person-years for those aged >65 years) in Rochester, Minn. [16], and 1.1 per 1,000 person-years in Seal Beach, Californian community [11], where the incidence of all strokes and TIA with previous cerebrovascular events were 7.1 and 1.4 per 1,000 person-years during the period 1963–1967, respectively.

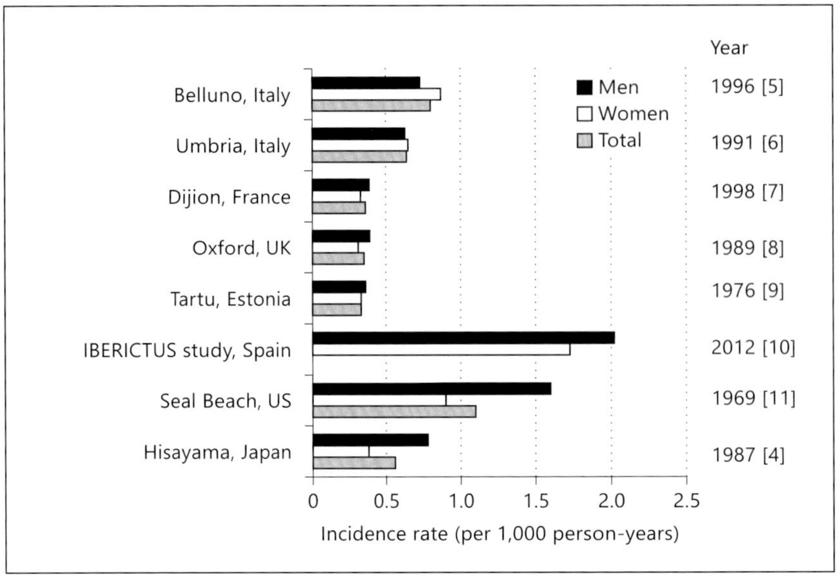

Fig. 1. Incidence of TIA in several countries.

The incidence for men was 9.7, 1.7 times the incidence of 5.7 for women per 1,000 person-years.

The incidence rate of TIA in Belluno, Italy, was 0.80 per 1,000 person-years, and the incidence was non-significantly higher in women than in men (0.73 per 1,000, 95% confidence interval, CI: 0.57–0.91 in men, and 0.87 per 1,000, 95% CI: 0.70–1.06 in women) [5]. After adjustment for the European population, the overall incidence rate decreased to 0.58 per 1,000 inhabitants per year. The mean age of new TIA patients was 73.9 years, and the women were significantly older than the men ($p < 0.001$). The SEPIVAC study of a population in Umbria, Italy revealed a crude rate of 0.64 per 1,000 per year (95% CI: 0.52–0.78), and the authors reported that the rate adjusted to the European population is 0.42 (95% CI: 0.33–0.54) [6]. It is of note that in the Umbria population, one third of the new TIA patients was cared for at home [6]. In Tartu, Estonia, USSR, from 1970 to 1973, the incidence of TIA was 0.33 per 1,000 person-years [9], and the mortality rate for stroke for this population was 0.98 per 1,000 person-years [9]. The Italian and Estonian data on the incidence of TIA, its dependence on age and sex, and mortality rate are close to the corresponding data reported from other countries.

The Oxfordshire Community Stroke Project showed that the crude TIA incidence rate and the TIA rate standardized to the 1981 population of England and Wales were 0.35 and 0.42 per 1,000 person-years, respectively [8]. The incidence of TIA increased sharply with increasing age, and the overall incidence in men was very similar to that

Table 2. Incidence and mortality of TIA according to age, sex, and race/ethnic group (per 1,000 person-years)

a Asia: Hisayama, Japan

Age group	Incidence		
	men	women	total
40–49 years	0.41	0.00	0.18
50–59 years	1.16	0.57	0.84
60–69 years	0.89	0.52	0.69
70– years	0.45	0.66	0.66
Total	0.78	0.38	0.56

b Europe

Age group	Incidence			Mortality		
	men	women	total	men	women	total
Udine District, Italy [5], 2007–2009						
<45 years	0.03	0.01	0.02			
45–54 years	0.29	0.05	0.16			
55–64 years	0.52	0.05	0.26			
65–74 years	0.94	0.71	0.81			
75–84 years	3.93	2.51	3.04			
85– years	5.34	3.44	3.95			
Total	0.56	0.49	0.52			
IBERICTUS, Spain [7]						
18–24 years	0.03	0.03	0.03	0.00	0.00	0.00
25–34 years	0.08	0.09	0.08	0.00	0.00	0.00
35–44 years	0.35	0.22	0.29	0.06	0.03	0.05
45–54 years	0.96	0.36	0.66	0.07	0.13	0.09
55–64 years	2.37	1.14	1.75	0.10	0.10	0.10
65–74 years	4.91	2.58	3.67	0.06	0.12	0.09
75–84 years	10.13	6.93	8.27	0.13	0.08	0.10
85– years	14.45	13.60	13.88	0.22	0.20	0.02
Total	2.02	1.73	1.87	0.11	0.12	0.12
Central Spain (the NEDICES study) [7]						
65–69 years	9.47	3.29	6.06			
70–74 years	11.27	15.25	13.49			
75–79 years	22.33	18.02	19.83			
80–84 years	10.75	15.22	13.53			
85– years	30.61	21.47	24.90			
Total	14.30	12.83	13.45			
Belluno, Italy [8]						
0–54 years	0.06	0.01	0.03			
55–64 years	1.09	1.04	1.06			
65–74 years	3.39	1.47	2.24			
75–84 years	7.20	6.06	6.39			
85– years	7.57	10.54	10.06			
Total	0.73	0.87	0.80			

Table 2. Continued

b Europe

Age group	Incidence			Mortality		
	men	women	total	men	women	total
Dijon, France [10]						
<34 years	0.00	0.01				
35–44 years	0.08	0.02				
45–54 years	0.27	0.00				
55–64 years	0.27	0.33				
65–74 years	1.50	1.03				
75–84 years	3.04	2.18				
85– years	4.68	2.20				
Total	0.39	0.33				
Oxfordshire, UK [12]						
<15 years	0.00	0.00	0.00			
15–44 years	0.02	0.02	0.02			
45–54 years	0.25	0.26	0.25			
55–64 years	1.22	0.63	0.92			
65–74 years	2.43	0.90	1.61			
75–84 years	3.01	2.29	2.57			
85– years	0.70	2.87	2.32			
Total	0.39	0.31	0.35			

Novosibirsk, Russia [13]

Age group	Incidence, 1987–1988			Incidence, 1996–1997		
	men	women	total	men	women	total
<45 years	0.02	0.02	0.02	0.02	0.01	0.01
45–64 years	0.49	0.40	0.44	0.68	0.47	0.56
65–74 years	1.26	0.38	0.68	1.24	1.39	1.34
75– years	0.34	0.56	0.51	2.27	1.74	1.85
Total	0.17	0.15	0.16	0.25	0.32	0.29

c America: Greater Cincinnati, Ohio [15]

Age group	Incidence (White)			Incidence (Black)		
	men	women	total	men	women	total
<35 years	0.01	0.02	–	0.02	0.03	–
35–44 years	0.05	0.12	–	0.16	0.13	–
45–54 years	0.85	0.72	–	1.30	0.30	–
55–64 years	1.55	0.96	–	2.06	2.49	–
65–74 years	4.68	2.47	–	3.38	3.30	–
75–84 years	7.5	5.21	–	6.13	6.47	–
85– years	7.19	5.89	–	15.60	8.47	–
Total	1.01	0.68	–	1.07	0.93	–

in women (incidence ratio 1.3). However, in middle age, men were 2.6 times more likely to suffer a TIA.

In Dijon, France, crude TIA incidence rates of 0.39 and 0.33 per 1,000 person-years were revealed for men and women, respectively [7]. The mean age of first-ever TIA was higher in women (71.8 years) than in men (70.4 years). CT scans were performed in 97% of the cases. These incidence rates were similar to those of previous population-based studies, such as Belluno [5], Tartu [9], and Oxford [8].

The IBERICTUS study results published in 2006 (2,257 strokes and 443 TIAs in patients aged >17 years) demonstrated that the incidence rates for the first TIA were 2.02 and 1.73 per 1,000 person-years in men and women [10], respectively, which are relatively higher than those in Japan. The IBERICTUS age-standardized (to the European population) incidence rates of TIA were 0.30 and 0.27, and those of all strokes (non-TIA) were 1.6 and 1.3 per 1,000 person-years in men and women, respectively; those of ischemic stroke were 4 times that of TIA and approximately one quarter that of intracerebral hemorrhage [10]. In addition, the in-hospital mortality rate of TIA patients was 0.11 and 0.12 per 1,000 person-years in men and women, respectively. However, a limitation of this study was that it is very difficult to detect TIA when there has only been a very short duration of TIA symptoms.

The Greater Cincinnati/Northern Kentucky Stroke Study reported that the age-adjusted rate was significantly lower for white women than for all other race/gender groups [14]. The total incidences of TIA were 1.01 and 0.68 per 1,000 in white men and women, and 1.07 and 0.93 in black men and women, respectively. The highest incidence of TIA of any group was seen in the very elderly black men (15.6 events per 1,000 person-years). The incidence of TIA increased very markedly with age, regardless of race or gender.

Symptoms of Transient Ischemic Attack

The ARIC study of several US populations found that 46.6% of the patients experienced at least one sudden-onset symptom of TIA, with 12.9% receiving a final diagnosis of TIA. The most common symptom among the TIA sudden-onset symptoms was dizziness (35.9%), but only 1.2% of the patients with dizziness had a final diagnosis of TIA, for a prevalence of 0.4% in all patients [2].

The Risk Factors for Transient Ischemic Attack

The risk factors for TIA or stroke are the same as those for other vascular diseases, similar to heart attack (coronary artery disease) or peripheral vascular disease, which causes decreased blood flow to the legs. However, the evidence of risk factors for TIA

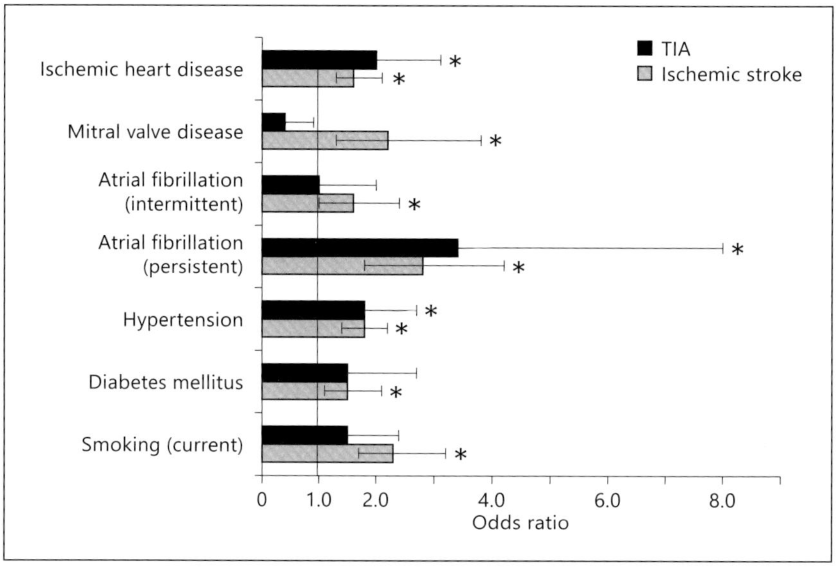

Fig. 2. Risk factors and their odds ratios for ischemic stroke and TIA.

excluding ischemic strokes has been very limited. In a case-control study from Mayo Clinic [16] odds ratios of strokes and TIA for various risk factors were calculated (fig. 2). For both ischemic heart disease and hypertension, the odds ratios of ischemic stroke were similar to those of TIA. Persistent and intermittent atrial fibrillations were found to be risk factors for ischemic stroke, while persistent atrial fibrillation was a risk factor only for TIA.

The Mayo Clinic data, which were collected over a 25-year period (1955–1979) show that TIA is a risk factor not only for stroke but also for death, especially death due to cardiovascular disease [16]. A 2010 meta-analysis revealed that there were no significant differences in sleep disorder breathing prevalence by event type, timing after stroke, or type of monitoring, although obstructive sleep apnea is very common in patients with TIA and stroke [17].

The ABCD score was developed to predict individuals at high early risk of stroke after TIA and to triage patients on the first presentation for medical attention [18]. The score is based on clinical characteristics detected at the time of first assessment for the following variables: Age ≥60 years, Blood pressure ≥140/90 mm Hg, Clinical features of TIA (weakness and speech impairment), and Duration of symptoms (≥60 or <60 min). This score was further validated and refined with the addition of a point for diabetes (ABCD^2 score) [19]. Details are described in the chapter by Wolf et al.

Prognosis of Stroke Events after Onset of Transient Ischemic Attack

Several risk scores have been developed to help stratify short-term stroke risk in patients with TIA [20]. The California score predicts the risk of stroke within 90 days. The ABCD score predicts the risk within 90 days and at 7 days, and the $ABCD^2$ score predicts the risk at 90, 30, 7, and 2 days.

A 2007 systematic review for early stroke risk after the onset of TIA demonstrated that the pooled stroke risks were 3.1 and 5.2% (95% CI: 2.0–4.1 and 3.9–6.5) at 2 and 7 days, respectively [21]. The lowest and highest risks were observed in studies of emergency treatment by stroke specialists (0.9%) and in population-based studies without emergency medications (11%), respectively.

There are very few studies on the long-term prognosis after the onset of TIA. A prospective study showed that the 10-year risks of stroke, myocardial infarction, and cardiovascular disease (stroke, myocardial infarction, or vascular death) were 18.8% (95% CI: 13.6–23.7), 27.8% (95% CI: 21.8–33.3), and 42.8% (95% CI: 36.4–48.5), respectively [22].

A review table shows prognosis stroke events after the onset of TIA according to race/ethnic group by time course (table 3) [14, 15, 17, 23–33]. A large study in Northern California noted that the 3-month stroke risk was 10.5% after the onset of TIA [31]. The risk of stroke after TIA in Canada was 9.5% at 3 months, and 14.5% at 1 year [26]. However, these studies were not performed with physician confirmation.

For many years, population-based data in Rochester have shown temporal trends in TIA incidence in the US [24]. However, black patients were only 1% of the Rochester study population, compared with 15.2% for the Greater Cincinnati/Northern Kentucky population mentioned earlier [14].

A meta-analysis of observational studies estimated the risk of stroke at 2, 30, and 90 days after TIA [34]. In that analysis, the pooled early risk of stroke was 3.5, 8.0, and 9.2% at 2, 30, and 90 days after TIA, respectively. This prognostic information is very valuable to patients and health care providers.

In the general population, the crude rates of stroke risk (%) were 1.7, 4.8, 6.6, 8.5, and 11.4 for 2 days, 1 week, 1 month, 3 and 6 months, respectively. In hospital patients, the rates were 13.7 and 12.4 for 1 and 3 months, respectively.

Family History

There is a very limited number of articles on the association between family history of stroke and the incidence of stroke after TIA. The Oxfordshire Community Stroke Project has shown that a family history of stroke does not predict the risk of ischemic stroke after TIA (odds ratio, 0.87; 95% CI: 0.57–1.32) [35]. Thus, the current available data show that the risk of ischemic stroke after TIA is not highly heritable.

Table 3. Prognosis of stroke events after onset of TIA according to race/ethnic groups

	Total	Stroke risk, %						Year and reference
		2 days	1 week	1 month	2 months	3 months	6 months	
General population								
Europe								
Rochester, Minn.	198			7.6		10.1		1973 [15]
Oxfordshire, UK	209		8.6	12.0				1990 [23] 2003 [24]
Southwest Germany	1,150						13.0	2004 [25]
America								
Nueces County, Tex.	612	1.6		3.2		4.0		2010 [17]
Alberta, Canada	2,285	1.4		6.7		9.5		2004 [26]
Greater Cincinnati, Ohio	927	2.4	3.9	6.9	7.8	8.6	9.5	2005 [14]
Crude averages		1.7	4.8	6.6		8.5	11.4	
Hospital-based population								
Europe								
London, UK	234						29.0	1981 [27]
Iowa City, Iowa	74		6.8[1]					1985 [28]
	62					8.1		1985 [28]
Oxford, UK	209			12.0				2003 [24]
Oxfordshire, UK	87			11.5		17.3		2004 [29]
Northern Portugal	141	9.9		17.7				2006 [30]
America								
Northern California	1,707					10.5		2000 [31]
Ontario, Canada	265					6.0		2004 [32]
NASCET	603					20.1		2004 [33]
Crude averages				13.7		12.4		

[1] Six days, 16.2% for recurrent TIA.

Diurnal and Seasonal Variations in Stroke and Transient Ischemic Attack Incidence

A seasonal variation in stroke incidence has been reported; increases in the stroke incidence, mortality, and the hospitalization of stroke patients during the winter season and a decrease during the warmer or summer seasons in the US [36] and Japan [37]. The Framingham Heart Study revealed that stroke events occurred significantly more often on Mondays than any other days, particularly for working men, and that during the day strokes occurred more frequently between 8 am and noon [36]. The Hisayama Study described a significant seasonality in the incidence of stroke subtypes (except for subarachnoid hemorrhage). In addition, the incidences of intracerebral hemorrhage and cerebral infarction were negatively associated with mean ambient temperature [37]. Karagiannis et al. [38] studying over 8,000 patients in a 10-year study in Greece, found that there was a significant seasonal variation for ischemic strokes with the average of 8.4% above peak incidence in spring and the average 10.4% below the lowest rate in summer.

The evidence for seasonal variations in TIA incidence is limited, in contrast to the many significant associations between stroke and seasonal variables. Manfredini et al. [39] showed that TIAs were most frequent in autumn and winter (the highest number of cases was in October), less common in spring and summer (the lowest number of cases was in February), and most frequent on Monday (all p values <0.0001). A large Hungarian registration study (n = 12,556) between 2005 and 2007 revealed that the peak period of TIA incidence was during spring (in May and April for men and women, respectively), whereas lowest number of events occurred in December for both sexes (p < 0.001), and that the highest morbidity from TIA occurred on Mondays for men and women [40]. There was no significant seasonal variation in the occurrence of intracerebral hemorrhage, subarachnoid hemorrhage, or TIA in northern Greece [38]. In a large stroke registry study in Japan (n = 12,660 patients), no seasonal difference was observed in stroke patients with a past history of stroke/TIA [41].

References

1 Pokorski RJ: Morbidity and mortality associated with transient ischemic attack (TIA). J Insur Med 1996;28:136–141.
2 Toole JF, Lefkowitz DS, Chambless LE, Wijnberg L, Paton CC, Heiss G: Self-reported transient ischemic attack and stroke symptoms: methods and baseline prevalence. The ARIC Study, 1987–1989. Am J Epidemiol 1996;144:849–856.
3 Karp HR, Heyman A, Heyden S, Bartel AG, Tyroler HA, Hames CG: Transient cerebral ischemia. Prevalence and prognosis in a biracial rural community. JAMA 1973;225:125–128.
4 Ueda K, Kiyohara Y, Hasuo Y, Yanai T, Kawano H, Wada J, Kato I, Kajiwara E, Omae T, Fujishima M: Transient cerebral ischemic attacks in a Japanese community, Hisayama, Japan. Stroke 1987;18:844–848.
5 Lauria G, Gentile M, Fassetta G, Casetta I, Agnoli F, Andreotta G, Barp C, Caneve G, Cavallaro A, Cielo R, Mongillo D, Mosca M, Olivieri P: Incidence of transient ischemic attacks in the Belluno Province, Italy. First-year results of a community-based study. Acta Neurol Scand 1996;93:291–296.
6 Ricci S, Celani MG, La Rosa F, Vitali R, Duca E, Ferraguzzi R, Paolotti M, Seppoloni D, Caputo N, Chiurulla C, et al: A community-based study of incidence, risk factors and outcome of transient ischaemic attacks in Umbria, Italy: the SEPIVAC study. J Neurol 1991;238:87–90.
7 Lemesle M, Madinier G, Menassa M, Billiar T, Becker F, Giroud M: Incidence of transient ischemic attacks in Dijon, France. A 5-year community-based study. Neuroepidemiology 1998;17:74–79.
8 Dennis MS, Bamford JM, Sandercock PA, Warlow CP: Incidence of transient ischemic attacks in Oxfordshire, England. Stroke 1989;20:333–339.
9 Zupping R, Roose M: Epidemiology of cerebrovascular disease in Tartu, Estonia, USSR, 1970 through 1973. Stroke 1976;7:187–190.
10 Diaz-Guzman J, Egido JA, Gabriel-Sanchez R, Barbera-Comes G, Fuentes-Gimeno B, Fernandez-Perez C: Stroke and transient ischemic attack incidence rate in Spain: The IBERICTUS Study. Cerebrovasc Dis 2012;34:272–281.
11 Friedman GD, Wilson WS, Mosier JM, Colandrea MA, Nichaman MZ: Transient ischemic attacks in a community. JAMA 1969;210:1428–1434.
12 Diaz-Guzman J, Bermejo-Pareja F, Benito-Leon J, Vega S, Gabriel R, Medrano MJ, Neurological Disorders in Central Spain Study G: Prevalence of stroke and transient ischemic attack in three elderly populations of central Spain. Neuroepidemiology 2008;30:247–253.

13 Feigin VL, Shishkin SV, Tzirkin GM, Vinogradova TE, Tarasov AV, Vinogradov SP, Nikitin YP: A population-based study of transient ischemic attack incidence in Novosibirsk, Russia, 1987–1988 and 1996–1997. Stroke 2000;31:9–13.

14 Kleindorfer D, Panagos P, Pancioli A, Khoury J, Kissela B, Woo D, Schneider A, Alwell K, Jauch E, Miller R, Moomaw C, Shukla R, Broderick JP: Incidence and short-term prognosis of transient ischemic attack in a population-based study. Stroke 2005;36:720–723.

15 Whisnant JP, Matsumoto N, Elveback LR: Transient cerebral ischemic attacks in a community. Rochester, Minnesota, 1955 through 1969. Mayo Clin Proc 1973;48:194–198.

16 Evans BA, Sicks JD, Whisnant JP: Factors affecting survival and occurrence of stroke in patients with transient ischemic attacks. Mayo Clin Proc 1994;69:416–421.

17 Johnson KG, Johnson DC: Frequency of sleep apnea in stroke and TIA patients: a meta-analysis. J Clin Sleep Med 2010;6:131–137.

18 Rothwell PM, Giles MF, Flossmann E, Lovelock CE, Redgrave JN, Warlow CP, Mehta Z: A simple score (ABCD) to identify individuals at high early risk of stroke after transient ischaemic attack. Lancet 2005;366:29–36.

19 Johnston SC, Rothwell PM, Nguyen-Huynh MN, Giles MF, Elkins JS, Bernstein AL, Sidney S: Validation and refinement of scores to predict very early stroke risk after transient ischaemic attack. Lancet 2007;369:283–292.

20 Purroy F, Begue R, Quilez A, Pinol-Ripoll G, Sanahuja J, Brieva L, Seto E, Gil MI: The California, ABCD, and unified ABCD2 risk scores and the presence of acute ischemic lesions on diffusion-weighted imaging in TIA patients. Stroke 2009;40:2229–2232.

21 Giles MF, Rothwell PM: Risk of stroke early after transient ischaemic attack: a systematic review and meta-analysis. Lancet Neurol 2007;6:1063–1072.

22 Clark TG, Murphy MF, Rothwell PM: Long term risks of stroke, myocardial infarction, and vascular death in 'low risk' patients with a non-recent transient ischaemic attack. J Neurol Neurosurg Psychiatry 2003;74:577–580.

23 Dennis M, Bamford J, Sandercock P, Warlow C: Prognosis of transient ischemic attacks in the Oxfordshire Community Stroke Project. Stroke 1990;21:848–853.

24 Lovett JK, Dennis MS, Sandercock PA, Bamford J, Warlow CP, Rothwell PM: Very early risk of stroke after a first transient ischemic attack. Stroke 2003;34:e138–e140.

25 Daffertshofer M, Mielke O, Pullwitt A, Felsenstein M, Hennerici M: Transient ischemic attacks are more than 'ministrokes'. Stroke 2004;35:2453–2458.

26 Hill MD, Yiannakoulias N, Jeerakathil T, Tu JV, Svenson LW, Schopflocher DP: The high risk of stroke immediately after transient ischemic attack: a population-based study. Neurology 2004;62:2015–2020.

27 Humphrey PR, Marshall J: Transient ischemic attacks and strokes with recovery prognosis and investigation. Stroke 1981;12:765–769.

28 Calandre L, Molina JA: Short-term outcome of medically treated patients with transient ischemic attacks, reversible ischemic neurologic deficits and strokes with minimum residuum. Eur Neurol 1985;24:281–285.

29 Coull AJ, Lovett JK, Rothwell PM, Oxford Vascular S: Population based study of early risk of stroke after transient ischaemic attack or minor stroke: implications for public education and organisation of services. BMJ 2004;328:326.

30 Correia M, Silva MR, Magalhaes R, Guimaraes L, Silva MC: Transient ischemic attacks in rural and urban northern Portugal: incidence and short-term prognosis. Stroke 2006;37:50–55.

31 Johnston SC, Gress DR, Browner WS, Sidney S: Short-term prognosis after emergency department diagnosis of TIA. JAMA 2000;284:2901–2906.

32 Gladstone DJ, Kapral MK, Fang J, Laupacis A, Tu JV: Management and outcomes of transient ischemic attacks in Ontario. CMAJ 2004;170:1099–1104.

33 Eliasziw M, Kennedy J, Hill MD, Buchan AM, Barnett HJ, North American Symptomatic Carotid Endarterectomy Trial G: Early risk of stroke after a transient ischemic attack in patients with internal carotid artery disease. CMAJ 2004;170:1105–1109.

34 Wu CM, McLaughlin K, Lorenzetti DL, Hill MD, Manns BJ, Ghali WA: Early risk of stroke after transient ischemic attack: a systematic review and meta-analysis. Arch Intern Med 2007;167:2417–2422.

35 Flossmann E, Rothwell PM: Family history of stroke does not predict risk of stroke after transient ischemic attack. Stroke 2006;37:544–546.

36 Kelly-Hayes M, Wolf PA, Kase CS, Brand FN, McGuirk JM, D'Agostino RB: Temporal patterns of stroke onset. The Framingham Study. Stroke 1995;26:1343–1347.

37 Shinkawa A, Ueda K, Hasuo Y, Kiyohara Y, Fujishima M: Seasonal variation in stroke incidence in Hisayama, Japan. Stroke 1990;21:1262–1267.

38 Karagiannis A, Tziomalos K, Mikhailidis DP, Semertzidis P, Kountana E, Kakafika AI, Pagourelias ED, Athyros VG: Seasonal variation in the occurrence of stroke in Northern Greece: a 10 year study in 8,204 patients. Neurol Res 2010;32:326–331.
39 Manfredini R, Manfredini F, Boari B, Malagoni AM, Gamberini S, Salmi R, Gallerani M: Temporal patterns of hospital admissions for transient ischemic attack: a retrospective population-based study in the Emilia-Romagna region of Italy. Clin Appl Thromb Hemost 2010;16:153–160.
40 Bodis J, Csoboth I, Gazdag L, Kriszbacher I: Seasonal variation, weekly and daily rhythm of transient ischemic attack in Hungary. Clin Appl Thromb Hemost 2010;16:232.
41 Ogata T, Kimura K, Minematsu K, Kazui S, Yamaguchi T, Japan Multicenter Stroke Investigators C: Variation in ischemic stroke frequency in Japan by season and by other variables. J Neurol Sci 2004;225: 85–89.

Yoshihiro Kokubo, MD, PhD, FAHA, FACC, FESC
Department of Preventive Cardiology
National Cerebral and Cardiovascular Center
5-7-1 Fujishiro-dai, Suita, Osaka 565-8565 (Japan)
E-Mail ykokubo@hsp.ncvc.go.jp

Uchiyama S, Amarenco P, Minematsu K, Wong KSL (eds): TIA as Acute Cerebrovascular Syndrome.
Front Neurol Neurosci. Basel, Karger, 2014, vol 33, pp 82–102 (DOI: 10.1159/000351905)

Symptoms of Transient Ischemic Attack

Jong S. Kim

Stroke Center and Department of Neurology, University of Ulsan, Asan Medical Center, Seoul, South Korea

Abstract

Transient ischemic attack (TIA) is a cerebrovascular disease with temporary (<24 h) neurological symptoms. The symptoms of TIA patients are largely similar to those of ischemic stroke patients and include unilateral limb weakness, speech disturbances, sensory symptoms, visual disturbances, and gait difficulties. As these symptoms are transient, they are frequently evaluated based on patients' subjective reports, which are less precise than those of patients with stroke whose longer-lasting symptoms and signs can be reliably assessed by physicians. Some symptoms, such as monocular blindness, are much more common in TIA than in stroke, and limb shaking occurs almost exclusively in TIA patients. On the other hand, symptoms like hemivisual field defects or limb ataxia are underappreciated in TIA patients. These transient neurological symptoms are not necessarily caused by cerebrovascular diseases, but can be produced by a variety of non-vascular diseases. Careful history taking, examination, and appropriate imaging tests are needed to differentiate these TIA mimics from TIA. Each TIA symptom has a different specificity and sensitivity, and there has been an effort to assess the outcome of the patients through the use of specific clinical features. On top of this, recent developments in imaging techniques have greatly enhanced our ability to predict the outcomes of TIA patients. Perception or recognition of TIA symptoms may differ according to the race, sex, education, and specialty of physicians. Appropriate education of both the general population and physicians with regard to TIA symptoms is important as TIAs need emergent evaluation and treatment.

Transient ischemic attack (TIA) is a cerebrovascular disease with temporary (<24 h) neurological symptoms. As the symptoms are transient, patients are frequently evaluated based on their subjective reports, which are less precise than those of stroke patients who are assessed by physicians in the presence of their symptoms/signs. While certain symptoms, such as hemivisual field loss or limb ataxia, are underappreciated, other symptoms, such as monocular blindness or limb shaking, occur much more frequently, or even exclusively, in TIA patients. Therefore, differences remain in the prevalence and characteristics of symptoms between TIA and stroke.

Table 1 lists the frequency of TIA symptoms in recent major studies [1–28]. Of these, unilateral motor symptoms are the most frequent, followed by speech disturbances and sensory symptoms. In this chapter, these symptoms will be described in detail. The sensitivity and specificity of these symptoms, TIA mimics, and problems in the perception and recognition of TIA symptoms will also be discussed.

Transient Ischemic Attack Symptoms

Hemiparesis and Other Types of Motor Dysfunction

As in patients with stroke, motor dysfunction is the most common manifestation of TIA (table 1). The most frequently observed topography is a weakness involving the arm, leg and face. The severity varies from severe, such as a complete inability to use limbs, to a subtle clumsiness of the hand or fingers. Although mild symptoms are more common in TIA patients, repeated occurrence of motor TIAs should be taken seriously because patients may eventually develop infarcts associated with severe motor dysfunction [29].

The somatic motor symptoms are usually attributed to the transient dysfunction of the pyramidal tract due to ischemic insult. However, because the symptom usually has disappeared or improved by the time the patient is seen by a physician, the underlying neurological problems are often difficult to correctly assess. It should be borne in mind that a subjective 'weakness' in the limbs may also be caused by dysfunction in the sensory (usually proprioceptive), coordination or extrapyramidal systems. Accordingly, the prevalence of 'motor dysfunction' in TIA patients is likely to be exaggerated. Moreover, even if patients only report motor problems, it does not necessarily mean that they did not have other neurological dysfunctions. For example, when tested in the emergency department, patients occasionally show decreased sensory perception in paralytic limbs that they had previously not noticed.

As in patients with stroke, topography involving the face, arm and leg together on one side is the most common. However, focal embolic ischemic events in the small area of the motor cortex may produce isolated weakness in the arm or the face, while involvement of a more medial part (i.e. the anterior cerebral artery territory) may produce weakness limited to the leg or the foot (fig. 1). In clinical practice, even if patients have hemiparesis involving the face, arm and the leg, they may recognize weakness in only a part of the body according to their situation when the symptoms occur. For example, patients who develop TIA while walking may report that they had symptoms only in the leg, whereas patients may only report arm weakness if the TIA develops while they are sitting down and using their arms.

Occasionally, patients complain of bilateral weakness. As this may be attributed to a severe vertebrobasilar disease, the accompanying symptoms and signs, such as dizziness, vertigo, diplopia or visual dimness, should be carefully examined. Severe, bilateral steno-occlusive disease in the anterior circulation may also produce bilateral

Table 1. Frequency of TIA symptoms in recent major studies

	Patients	Ethnicity	Symptom assessment	Motor symptom %	Speech disturbance %	Sensory symptoms %	Vertebrobasilar symptoms, %	Gait disturbance, %
Johnston et al. [1]	1,707	US (80% White)	PCP	45.9	42.2	40.0	36.6	25.1
Rothwell et al. [2]								
OCSP	209	UK	N	53.5	12.4			
OXVASC	190	UK	N	49.4	22.1			
OXVASC	378	UK	PCP	31.2	19.3			
Hospital clinic	210	UK	PCP	37.6	21.4			
Johnston et al. [3]								
California ED	1,069	US (70% White)	PCP	44.1	35.8			
California clinic	962	US (70% White)	PCP	33.4	25.4			
Oxford population-based	547	UK (95% White)	PCP	30.5	31.2			
Oxford clinic	315	UK (94% White)	PCP	35.5	35.8			
Bray et al. [4]	98	Australian	PCP	57.1	19.3			
Calvet et al. [5]	343	French	PCP	47.8	22.4			
Perry et al. [6]	2,056	Canadian	PCP	43.7	37.5	45.3	12.2	22.7
Al-Khaled et al. [7]	1,862	German	PCP, N	25.4	25.6			
Cucchiara et al. [8]	117	US	N	35.8	23.9			
Tsivgoulis et al. [9]	226	Greek	N	46.5	42.5	37.6	11.9	5.8
Lavallée et al. [10]	643	French	SN	38.7	37.3			
Purroy et al. [11]	388	Spanish	N	46.1	33.2			
Park et al. [12]	98	Korean	N	73.4	48.9	11.2		
Sciolla et al. [13]	274	Italian	N	58.0	25.5			
Coutts et al. [14]	180	Canadian	SN	81.6	18.3			
Amarenco et al. [15]	1,176	French	SN	36.6	37.9	24.0	29.3	
Ay et al. [16]	477	US	N	47.4	56.0			
Sheehan et al. [17]	292	Irish	SN	52.7	23.6			
Tsivgoulis et al. [18]	148	59% White 41% Asian	N	34.4	35.8	46.6	16.2	4.7
Nakajima et al. [19]	133	Japanese	N	69.9	51.3	22.1	18.5	58.4
Meng et al. [20]	410	Chinese	N	58.7	7.0			
von Weitzel-Mudersbach et al. [21]	306	Danish	N	44.8	22.2	8.8	12.4	
Amort et al. [22]	248	Swiss	SN	58.5	42.0	34.3	34.6	
Cancelli et al. [23]	161	Italian	N	44.7	35.4			
Poisson et al. [24]	97	US (90% White)	SN	55.6	28.8			
Purroy et al. [25]	1,137	Spanish	N	58.7	64.6	7.7	12.0	
Coutts et al. [26]	499	Canadian	SN	64.1	30.6			
Dolatabadi et al. [27]	150	Farsi	N	48.0	38.7			
Hoshino et al. [28]	133	Japanese	SN	59.4	21.1			

PCP = Primary care physician, which includes generalists, internists, family doctors, and emergency department physicians; N = neurologist; SN = stroke neurologist.
Vertebrobasilar symptoms indicate dizziness, vertigo, ataxia, and visual symptoms.

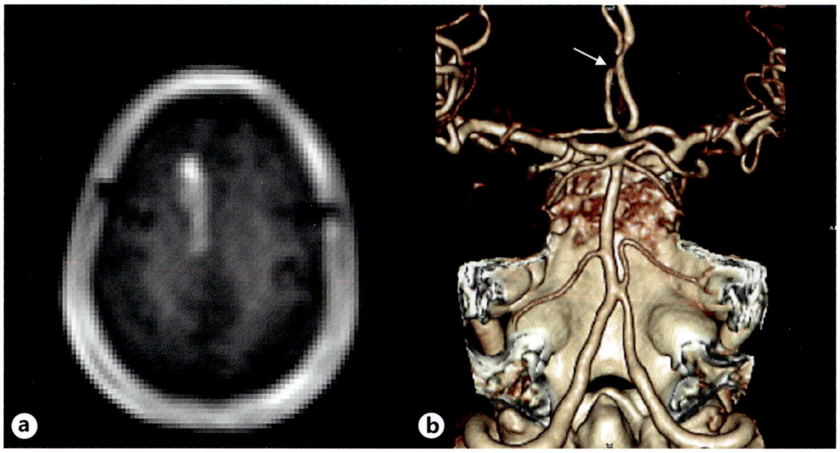

Fig. 1. A 79-year-old hypertensive woman developed weakness on the left leg lasting <1 min, when she could not walk and had to sit down for a while. The episodes occurred approximately once a day. One month later, she developed prolonged left leg weakness associated with dysarthria and urinary incontinence. DWI showed an acute infarction in the right anterior cerebral artery territory (**a**), and CT angiography showed severe focal stenosis on the right anterior cerebral artery (arrow; **b**).

weakness. In clinical practice, this symptom is more often associated with unilateral cerebrovascular diseases of the anterior circulation; the presence of uncrossed pyramidal fibers may partly explain this phenomenon. In addition, patients may perceive sudden gait impairment as bilateral leg weakness when it is actually due to unilateral weakness.

There are patients who show repeated, stereotyped motor (or occasionally sensorimotor) hemiparesis involving the face, arm and leg simultaneously with no cortical signs such as aphasia or neglect. This is often described as 'capsular warning syndrome' because the affected region is probably the subcortical area (i.e., internal capsule) or, less often, the pontine base [29, 30]. The presumed mechanism is a repeated hemodynamic compromise in penetrating vessels associated with thrombosis within the penetrating artery or at the stenotic portion of parental vessels (middle cerebral artery or basilar artery). Although capsular warning syndrome is uncommon (1.5–4.5% of TIA patients), physicians should be alert for this condition because symptomatic or asymptomatic infarcts in the internal capsule/basal ganglia or the pontine base occur in as many as 42–60% of these patients [29, 31] (fig. 2).

Somatosensory Symptoms

Sensory symptoms/signs occur in more than half of stroke patients. However, sensory symptoms as a manifestation of TIA are less common (table 1). This is because patients usually notice the symptoms only when they are positive (e.g. tingling, numb). Although patients may discover that they do not feel as expected when their body

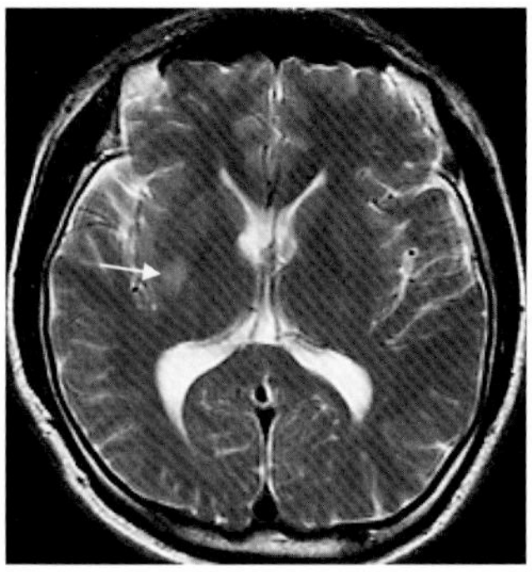

Fig. 2. A 41-year-old hypertensive man suddenly developed recurrent left hemiparesis involving arm, leg and face, and dysarthria that lasted for about 10 min. The episodes recurred 5 times. Neurological examination findings were normal. T2-weighted brain MRI showed a small infarct involving the right putamen and internal capsule (arrow). Transfemoral angiogram findings were normal.

parts are in contact with objects (e.g. a spoon, bar or wheel), it is rare to see patients visit emergency departments with this problem as a chief complaint.

In patients with ischemic stroke, motor dysfunction is often associated with a concomitant decrease in sensory perception in the involved limbs. This is probably the same in TIA patients, but patients simply do not recognize this and thus report the symptom as a pure limb weakness. Moreover, as discussed above, positional or discriminatory sensory disturbances may be perceived by the patients as a 'weakness' of the limbs. For these reasons, it is likely that sensory dysfunction in TIA patients is underappreciated.

On the other hand, sensory symptoms are one of the least specific symptoms of TIA (see below). A transient numb, tingling or painful sensation in the limbs may be a symptom of radiculopathy or peripheral neuropathy. Moreover, these also are manifestations of anxiety or hysteria. Hysterical or conversion neurosis should be suspected when the patient is young and does not have vascular risk factors. The patients usually have additional, even multiple, somatic complaints, and do not sufficiently focus on sensory symptoms. Moreover, the distribution of the sensory dysfunction may not fit with the usual clinical pattern (e.g. bilateral hand or feet numbness), although sensory symptoms in the hemibody distribution are also occasionally observed in neurotic patients.

As in stroke patients, sensory TIA is usually accompanied by other neurological symptoms, such as motor dysfunction, and 'pure' sensory TIA is uncommon. In 1982, Fisher [32] described 42 patients with pure sensory TIA, in whom the face, arm and leg were involved in 33 (79%), the face and arm in 3 (7%), the arm and leg in 4 (9%), and only the face in 2 (5%) patients. Pathological findings in one patient showed a lateral thalamic infarction. More recently, Kim [33] described patients with repeated, pure sensory TIAs with or without posterior cerebral artery stenosis. The presumed mechanism is repeated hemodynamic compromise of the thalamogeniculate artery in the presence of thrombus within the perforating artery or at the stenotic portion of the posterior cerebral artery. These patients may or may not develop eventual lateral thalamic infarction. Accordingly, this phenomenon is considered a sensory counter-

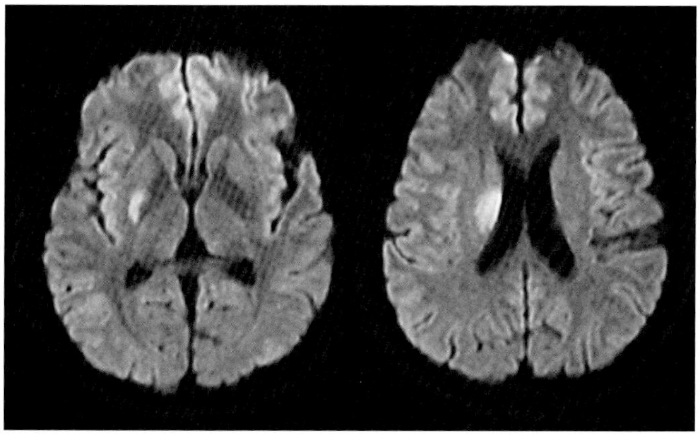

Fig. 3. A 42-year-old hypertensive man suddenly developed two episodes of dysarthria lasting about 20 min each, without any difficulty in walking or using his arms. Neurological examination results were normal. DWI showed an infarct involving the putamen and the genu portion of the internal capsule.

part of capsular warning syndrome. In addition, the author has observed patients who developed occipital infarcts following sensory TIAs associated with posterior cerebral artery stenosis, which may be related to an eventual development of an artery-to-artery embolism arising from the atherosclerotic posterior cerebral artery diseases. Nonetheless, pure sensory TIAs are not necessarily caused by posterior circulation diseases. Recurrent sensory TIAs are occasionally observed in patients with middle cerebral artery atherosclerosis, which may even herald a large middle cerebral artery territory infarction [34].

Finally, there are patients who report tingling sensations restricted to bilateral perioral or tongue tip areas. Although this sensory distribution is not specific for posterior circulation diseases, one should be alert on this symptom because it may reflect a significant basilar artery disease, potentially heralding catastrophic brainstem strokes [35].

Speech Disturbances

Speech disturbances are another relatively frequent TIA symptom (table 1) attributed to dysarthria and/or aphasia.

Dysarthria

In TIA patients, dysarthria is usually associated with a motor dysfunction in the extremities or the face. It can be produced by ischemic events occurring on either side of the anterior hemisphere as well as in the posterior circulation. Dysarthria is generally attributed to the involvement of the corticobulbar tract, but it can also be caused by extrapyramidal or cerebellar system dysfunction. Therefore, dysarthria has no localizing value. In addition, it is occasionally difficult to differentiate dysarthria from motor aphasia by history alone. Although uncommon, patients with episodes of lone dysarthria are observed who suffer selective ischemic damage on the corticobulbar tract (i.e. the genu portion of the internal capsule; fig. 3).

Aphasia

As in stroke patients, aphasia in TIA patients can manifest as global, motor or sensory aphasia. In clinical practice, symptoms suggesting motor aphasia (inability to speak) are much more common than sensory aphasia (inability to understand). This is at least in part attributed to the difficulty in differentiating motor aphasia from dysarthria. Moreover, unlike problems that occur during active speaking, limitation in understanding is not well appreciated by the patients unless they are involved in prolonged conversation. Therefore, even if patients report that they did not have particular difficulty in understanding others, it is not clear whether the patients are without sensory aphasia unless they are examined by a physician at the time of the episode. Other types of aphasia, such as transcortical or conduction aphasia, are extremely difficult to detect. Occasionally, patients report that they had difficulty recalling names or words, but again it remains uncertain whether they had purely anomic aphasia by history taking alone.

As aphasia is generally caused by left-sided brain damage, the presence of arterial (internal carotid or middle cerebral artery) disease on the left side more convincingly suggests that the patients' speech disturbances were due to aphasia. These patients may experience right hemiparesis/hemisensory disturbances preceding, following or at the time of the aphasic episodes. As aphasia is a cortical symptom, it is not observed in capsular or small vessel disease-associated TIA. One study showed that TIA patients with atrial fibrillation more often present with aphasia than those without [36].

Dysphagia

Dysphagia is caused by ischemic damage on the corticobulbar tracts or the nucleus ambiguus and related structures in the brain stem. Therefore, dysphagia is almost always accompanied by dysarthria or other brain stem symptoms. Because dysphagia is often mild or even absent in patients with unilateral corticobulbar tract dysfunction, dysphagia as a symptom of TIA is less common than dysarthria. Furthermore, dysphagia can manifest only when patients eat or drink something, and is therefore less likely to be detected by patients. For these reasons, TIA patients presenting with isolated dysphagia are extremely rare.

Visual Symptoms

Monocular Blindness

Transient monocular blindness (TMB) refers to sudden, brief attacks of partial or complete dimness or obscuration of vision. The term 'amaurosis fugax' has been used interchangeably, but not without confusion [37], and TMB, a less controversial term, will be used in this chapter. TMB episodes typically last seconds or minutes. Patients may report that they have complete blindness when the other eye is covered. More often, patients report partial symptoms variably described as 'things look suddenly gray', 'margins of items become blurred' or 'curtains are ascending

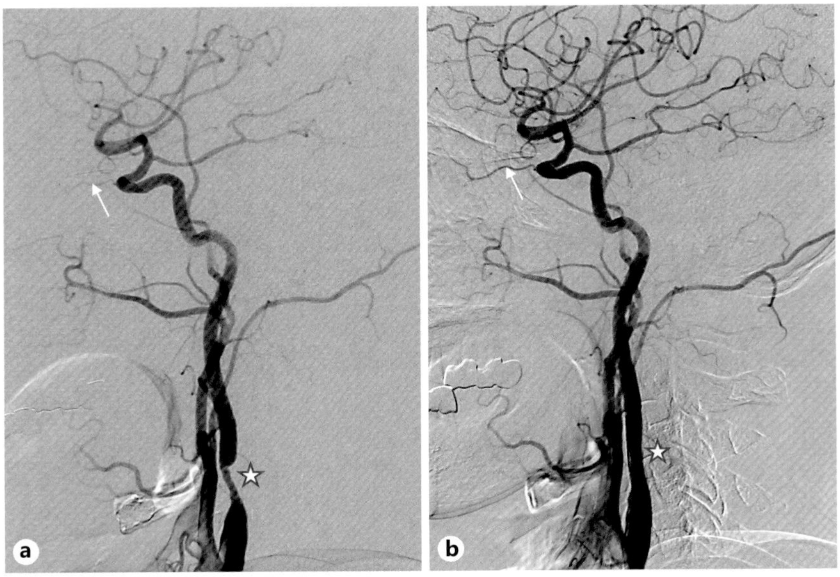

Fig. 4. A 67-year-old hypertensive and diabetic man developed brief episodes of right visual obscuration lasting 1 or 2 min. Brain MRI showed normal findings. **a** Conventional angiography showed severe stenosis in the proximal internal carotid artery (star) and reduced blood flow in the ophthalmic artery (arrow). **b** After the stenting procedure, there was improvement of the carotid stenosis and ophthalmic artery flow. The episodes of visual dimness no longer developed afterwards.

or descending', or as a gradual shading from the periphery to the center in the affected visual field. Dimming of vision may occur in the upper or lower half of the visual field. Less commonly, scintillations or other positive visual phenomena may occur.

TMB is usually associated with significant carotid atherosclerotic stenosis/occlusion (fig. 4) and occasionally co-occurs with contralateral hemiparesis [38]. Although carotid disease at the bulb area has traditionally been described as the cause of TMB, TMB caused by distal (usually cavernous portion) internal carotid artery disease is occasionally observed in Asia where intracranial atherosclerosis is prevalent.

Transient embolic occlusion of the ophthalmic artery, central retinal artery or the posterior ciliary arteries secondary to the detachment of platelets or cholesterol crystals from ulcerated plaques seems to cause TMB. Ophthalmic examination may show an occlusion of retinal arteries by cholesterol crystals (Hollenhorst plaques) or platelet-fibrin. However, normal ophthalmic examination findings at the time of TMB do not necessarily indicate the absence of embolic material. The symptoms are often associated with hemodynamically unstable conditions such as dehydration, sudden standing, and exhaustion, and angiographic studies frequently reveal decreased perfusion in the ophthalmic artery (fig. 4). Therefore, periodic reduction in ophthalmic artery blood flow seems to play an additional role in TMB.

Regardless of the presence of TMB episodes, the presence of retinal emboli predicts higher all-cause and stroke-related mortality than in patients without these findings. In patients who show cholesterol embolus in the retina, the annual mortality rate is four to five times greater than in those without, with the most frequent cause of death being either coronary heart disease [39] or stroke [40].

In some patients, TMB occurs less rapidly, lasts longer (minutes to hours), and ameliorates more gradually (sometimes called TMB type II). Typically, patients' visual symptoms occur when they are exposed to bright light [41]. Rather than perceiving a significant decrease in visual acuity, patients describe that bright objects appear brighter and more dazzling, so that they have difficulty in seeing objects clearly. They often cannot read letters written on white papers.

These symptoms are associated with very severe carotid stenosis or complete occlusion. The episodes are preceded by hypotension, exhaustion, and conditions associated with increased venous pressure such as stooping or straining or a warm environment. Temporarily lowered retinal artery pressure secondary to severe carotid hypoperfusion and diversion of blood to the external carotid artery system is considered a likely mechanism. Ophthalmic examination shows lowered retinal artery pressure and occasional retinal venous stasis. Aggravated symptoms upon light exposure may be explained by the inability of borderline circulation to sustain the increased retinal metabolic activity associated with light exposure or delayed regeneration of visual pigments in the pigment epithelial layer. Bilateral visual loss associated with severe bilateral carotid occlusive disease has also been reported [42].

In addition to carotid atherosclerosis, TMB may be caused by carotid artery dissection, atherosclerosis on the aorta, and arteritis (such as giant cell arteritis and Takayasu disease). Embolism from heart disease, a systemic coagulopathy (e.g. polycythemia vera), leukemia, and antiphospholipid antibody syndrome may also be associated with TMB.

Finally, some patients show repeated TMB but without any evidence of carotid disease or other embolic sources. In at least some of these patients, retinal or ophthalmic artery vasospasm seems to be the cause of the TMB (TMB type III) [43]. In this group of patients, the visual loss attacks tend to be frequent, recurring many times a day. The patients often have temporary complete monocular blindness rather than visual loss restricted to the inferior or superior altitudinal field. Some patients experience a prodromal ocular aching before losing their vision. Medical histories of these patients may reveal migraine, Raynaud's disease, systemic lupus erythematosus, and other conditions causing hypercoagulability or vasospasm. Thus, patients with this 'vasospastic' TMB may comprise two groups: young (<50-year-old) patients with a history of migraine, autoimmune diseases, etc. and older patients without. Ophthalmic examination at the time of TMB may show multiple constriction of retinal arterioles and rouleaux formation in venules, indicating vasospasm and sluggish blood flow. Identifying this group of patients is important because they may respond to calcium channel blockers and not antithrombotics [43].

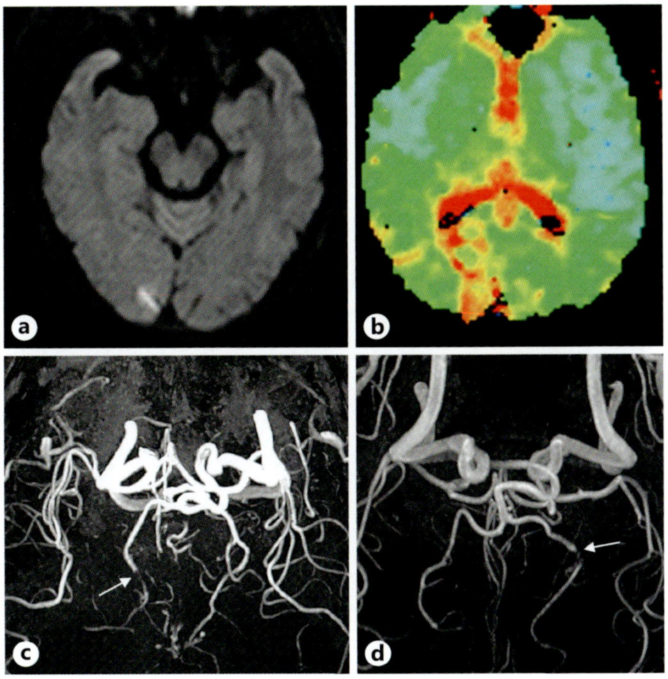

Fig. 5. A 78-year-old hypertensive woman suddenly could not clearly see television and people around her. She reported that there was general dimness in vision although she could recognize people and color. However, she did not attempt to cover one eye during the episode. The episode recurred several times a day, and 2 days later, when she visited our clinic, neurologic examination revealed left hemianopia. Diffusion- and perfusion-weighted MRIs showed a small infarct (**a**) and decreased perfusion (**b**) in the right occipital area. **c** MR angiogram showed a focal severe stenosis in the right posterior cerebral artery (arrow). A 72-year-old hypertensive and hypercholesterolemic woman suddenly experienced visual obscuration on the right side that lasted about 10 min. The episodes recurred about once in a few days. During these episodes, she attempted to cover the right or the left eye, and found that the visual symptom remained identical. Neurologic examination findings were normal. Brain MRI was normal. **d** MR angiogram showed a focal stenosis on the P2 portion of the left posterior cerebral artery (arrow).

Hemivisual Field Defects

Hemivisual field defects (hemianopia or quadrantanopia) are an uncommon TIA symptom, partly because a transient visual field defect frequently goes unnoticed by patients, and partly because patients often do not correctly notice that their problem is a hemivisual field defect; patients may report that they have a visual problem on the entire field (fig. 5a–c) or on their one eye, thus making it difficult to be differentiated from bilateral visual field disturbances or TMB. Only occasionally will patients try at the time of symptom onset to cover one eye to determine whether their symptoms are a visual field defect or TMB (fig. 5d). According to one study where all the TIA patients were examined by perimetry, asymptomatic visual field defects were found in

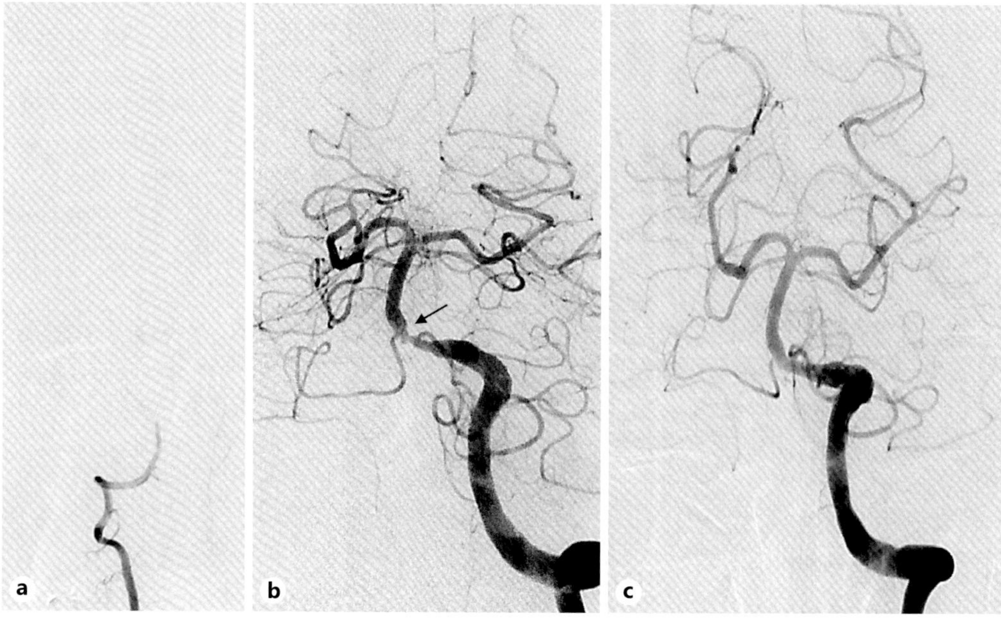

Fig. 6. A 65-year-old hypertensive man with congestive heart failure developed dizziness and bilateral visual dimness especially when he walked on a sunny day, which improved on rest in 1 or 2 min. Occasionally, dizziness was associated with perioral and tongue tip tingling sensation, which was followed by dysarthria, and quadriparesis. The episodes lasted 5–10 min, and developed once or a few times a day, usually at the time when the patient was exhausted. Brain MRI findings were normal. Conventional angiogram showed occlusion of the distal portion of the hypoplastic right vertebral artery (**a**) and severe stenosis in the distal part of the left vertebral artery (arrow; **b**). **c** After angioplasty and stenting, there was improvement in the stenosis, and his symptoms no longer developed.

as many as 29% of patients, predominantly located in the upper part of the visual field [44]. This result suggests that hemivisual field defects are actually more common in TIA patients than previously realized.

Bilateral Visual Blurring or Field Defects

Transient bilateral visual loss, an uncommon manifestation of TIA, may occur under several conditions. First, in patients who had previously suffered a stroke and a subsequent hemivisual field defect, the occurrence of another ischemic attack involving the contralateral occipital area may produce a bilateral visual field defect. More frequently, a transient bilateral visual field defect is caused by a sudden decrease in the perfusion of both occipital areas, attributed either to hypoperfusion or embolism, usually associated with severe vertebrobasilar occlusive diseases. The visual symptom is usually associated with concurrent symptoms of posterior circulation TIAs such as vertigo, ataxia, diplopia or quadriparesis (fig. 6). Finally, as discussed above, patients may complain of bilateral visual dimness when there actually are unilateral occipital ischemic events (fig. 5).

Bilateral visual field defects as the only symptom of TIA is rare. Recently, 6 patients who presented with transient (1–15 min), isolated bilateral blindness were reported [45]. The patients had vascular risk factors, and 2 of them suffered subsequent TIAs. The symptoms were therefore considered to be due to a TIA that affected the bilateral occipital areas, probably related to embolic events. However, only one patient had a severe basilar artery stenosis and one had atrial fibrillation. Transient bilateral visual field defects without any signs of posterior circulation symptoms should be differentiated from migraine.

Although less common, transient bilateral visual disturbances may be associated with severe bilateral carotid steno/occlusive diseases. Patients may develop more severe symptoms when they are exposed to light, which is apparently related to the delayed regeneration of visual pigments in the pigment epithelial layer associated with significant bilateral retinal ischemia [42]. Finally, bilateral visual obscuration may be a preceding or associated symptom of a sudden lowering of blood pressure or a syncopal attack, and these conditions should be differentiated from those of TIA.

Vertigo and Dizziness

Vertigo is a feeling that objects in the environment are spinning around or moving rhythmically. Patients may also feel that their heads or bodies are whirling. Vertigo is often associated with nausea, vomiting, and gait instability, and patients veer or appear to be pulled to one side (pulsion) while walking. Vertigo is an important symptom of TIA in the vertebrobasilar artery territory and is usually associated with other neurological symptoms such as dysarthria, diplopia, ataxia and visual disturbances. For isolated vertigo, however, TIA is definitely an uncommon cause. Much more common causes are otologic (or labyrinthine) diseases, including Ménière's disease, benign paroxysmal positional vertigo, toxic (such as drug-caused) vestibulopathy, and vestibular neuronitis. In addition, vertigo may be a symptom of seizures or migraines.

Of note, however, is the fact that small infarcts occurring in the medial part of the cerebellum (medial posterior inferior cerebellar artery territory), including the nodular area, may produce isolated vertigo without any other neurological abnormalities. The vertigo may be transient and even recurrent. Moreover, recent studies have reported that isolated vertigo is a relatively common symptom in patients who later develop vertebrobasilar territory stroke [46, 47]. Therefore, this possibility should also be kept in mind, especially if patients have vascular risk factors or a previous history of vascular diseases.

Non-vertiginous dizziness is distinguished from vertigo by the lack of feeling of rotation, impulsion or oscillopsia, and the rare occurrence of nausea, vomiting and gait imbalance. Dizziness is also a common symptom of TIA associated with vertebrobasilar artery steno/occlusive disease (fig. 6). However, dizziness is an extremely common symptom associated with a variety of clinical conditions such as orthostatic hypotension, presyncope, heart failure, arrhythmia, hypoglycemia, anxiety/depression, and the use of a variety of drugs. Recently, Kerber et al. [48] studied patients presenting with dizziness symptoms (including dizziness, vertigo and gait imbalance), and found that stroke/TIA was diagnosed in 3.2% (53 of 1,666) and that only 0.7% (9 of 1,297) of those with isolated symptoms had a stroke/TIA. Therefore, the proportion of cerebrovascular events in patients presenting with isolated dizziness symptoms seems to be very low.

Diplopia

Diplopia is a symptom of ocular motor dysfunction secondary to ischemic lesion in the brainstem. Accordingly, diplopia is usually associated with preceding or concomitant symptoms suggestive of posterior circulation disease, such as vertigo, dysarthria or ataxia.

Depending upon the dysfunctional ocular motor system, patients may report that diplopia is more prominent in certain conditions or when they look in certain directions. For instance, patients may have maximal diplopia on horizontal gaze when there is a 6th nerve palsy, whereas patients may report difficulty while stepping down a ladder if they have skew deviation or 4th nerve palsy. Some patients may describe dizziness or gait instability that improves while one eye is covered without specifically noticing diplopia.

It is very rare to see TIA patients who present with diplopia as a lone symptom. In this occasion, other causes should be more seriously considered, such as myasthenia gravis, ocular motor neuropathy, inflammatory cranial neuropathy, thyroid disease, and skull base tumor, although vertebrobasilar TIA should still not be excluded.

Ataxia

Limb incoordination (dysmetria), rate changes in voluntary movements, tremulous movements on action, and gait instability with veering to one side are symptoms indicating cerebellar dysfunction. These are important symptoms of posterior circulation TIAs, along with other symptoms such as vertigo and diplopia.

However, ataxia as a lone symptom is uncommon in TIA patients, as they often report this dysfunction as 'limb weakness', 'dizziness' or 'gait difficulty'. Likewise, slurred, scanning dysarthria due to cerebellar dysfunction can simply be reported as 'speech disturbances'. Thus, limb incoordination is likely to be underappreciated in TIA patients. Furthermore, even if patients describe their symptoms as 'incoordination', the symptoms may still be caused by motor or sensory dysfunction. Therefore, it is extremely difficult to assess whether the symptoms are truly associated with cerebellar dysfunction unless the symptoms are associated with other posterior circulation TIA symptoms or patients are examined by neurologists at the time of the TIA.

Loss of Consciousness or Syncope

Syncope is defined as a sudden transient loss of consciousness associated with an inability to maintain postural tone. Syncope is a common medical condition and many people who experience syncope worry about the possibility of cerebrovascular disease. However, TIA is a rare (1.5–2%) cause of syncope [49, 50]. More frequently, it is caused by cardiac arrhythmia, orthostatic hypotension, and vasovagal instability. Nevertheless, more recent larger studies reported that TIA may be a cause of syncope in up to 7.7% [51] or 11% [52] of patients. The syncopes in these patients are frequently accompanied by vertebrobasilar TIA symptoms such as vertigo and ataxia. Vertebrobasilar steno/occlusive diseases or, less commonly, bilateral carotid artery occlusive diseases, are often found. Therefore, the possibility of TIA should be borne in mind in syncopal patients with significant vascular risk factors and accompanying neurological symptoms/signs. The syncope in these patients seems to be attributed to an ischemia of the brainstem reticular activating structures responsible for the regulation of alertness and postural tone.

Headache

Headache, often associated with large strokes, especially hemorrhagic strokes, is generally considered a symptom that precludes TIA diagnosis (see below). However, a few studies focusing on this issue have reported that headache as a preceding or concomitant symptom of TIA is not uncommon, occurring in up to 24–30% of TIA patients [53, 54]. Headache seems to occur more often in females than in males and in patients with vertebrobasilar TIA than in those with carotid TIA. It is usually described as pulsating or throbbing, and less often, pressing, and of a mild to moderate degree. Headache tends to occur on the ipsilateral side of the TIA, in the anterior half of the head in the carotid TIA, and in the posterior half of the head in the vertebrobasilar TIA. However, approximately half of the patients have generalized or nonlocalizing headache, and there only is a weak correlation between the pain area and the TIA territory.

Headache in TIA patients may be related to vascular/cerebral damage, vasodilation of collateral arteries or anxiety associated with the sudden development of neurological dysfunction. The molecular mechanisms of headache in TIA may include release of nitric oxide from the ischemic brain or vessels and neurogenic inflammation in cerebral arteries (trigeminovascular system) mediated by a series of vasoactive neuropeptides (e.g., calcitonin gene-related peptide and substance P). The predominant ipsilateral distribution of the neuronal fibers explains the ipsilateral distribution of headache in many patients, whereas bilateral innervations of certain midline vessels, such as the sagittal sinus and the anterior cerebral arteries, may explain the bilateral distribution of headache in others. Infratentorial arteries, such as the basilar arteries, may have dual – trigeminal and cervical – innervation, which may implicate vertebrobasilar disease in frontal pain [55]. Although the presumed mechanism of headache in TIA resembles that of migraine, the presence of migraine prior to the ischemic event does not appear to increase susceptibility to TIA-related headaches.

Finally, arterial dissection causing TIA is undoubtedly an important cause of severe headache occurring in young patients.

Limb Shaking and Other Involuntary Movements

Episodic 'limb shaking' is a well-known TIA symptom that is uncontrollable, stereotypical, and lasts from seconds to minutes [56]. Occasionally, more complex symptoms, such as irregular wavering, flapping, circling or trembling movements, are observed. Symptoms are more often seen in the arm than in the leg, and tend to be elicited by sitting, standing or exhaustion. These symptoms are usually associated with severe carotid [56] or, less often, middle cerebral [57] or anterior cerebral artery [58] steno-occlusive diseases associated with significant hemodynamic impairments. The nature of the vascular lesion is most often atherosclerosis, but other pathologies such as dissection or moyamoya disease may also produce similar symptoms.

The term 'limb shaking' is easily understood by patients, and has been frequently used among physicians. However, this is not a strictly medical term and the precise pathogenic nature of limb shaking remains unclear. Although the phenomenon resembles focal motor seizures, electroencephalographic studies have failed to show the epileptiform activity associated with the symptoms. Perfusion studies have shown significant hypoperfusion of the border zone areas contralateral to the shaking limb, suggesting transient hemodynamic failure to be the cause of the symptoms. According to the author's observation, some patients with frontal lobe infarcts initially present with gross limb shaking that diminishes in intensity to become asterixis. Therefore, the limb shaking symptoms may be a severe form of asterixis in at least some of these patients [59]. Postural tone is under the control of cortico-subcortical pathways involving the basal ganglia, motor thalamus, cerebellum, and frontal-parietal neocortex, and hypoperfusion in the contralateral frontoparietal regions may lead to intermittent failure of postural control in these patients.

In addition, transient or persistent hemichorea may be caused by atherosclerosis or moyamoya-associated carotid artery disease, probably related to perfusion failure in the contralateral basal ganglia [60]. The author observed a patient with transient hemichorea associated with unilateral middle cerebral artery atherosclerotic disease.

Cognitive and Emotional Symptoms

Various cognitive or behavioral impairments, such as apathy, neglect, memory loss, apraxia, agraphia, and acalculia, are observed in stroke patients with cortical lesions or strategic subcortical lesions involving the capsular genu or the anterior thalamus. However, it is rare to see TIA patients presenting with these cognitive problems as a main complaint. This is partly because cognitive dysfunction may become apparent only when patients are exposed to sudden circumstances (e.g. acalculia may be detected by patients only when they are paying for something) and partly because the symptoms are not precisely identified and appropriately recognized as a serious vascular event by the patients.

Nevertheless, transient global amnesia (TGA), a condition characterized by transient, but significant, memory impairment deserves special attention. The etiology and pathogenesis of TGA remains obscure. Several different mechanisms such as seizure, migraine, venous congestion and vascular diseases, associated with consecutive damage at memory relevant structures, have been suggested. Generally, TGA has characteristics different from those of cerebrovascular diseases: patients are younger and have less frequent vascular risk factors, a low recurrence rate, and a better long-term outcome. However, recent reports have shown diffusion-weighted MRI (DWI)-positive lesions in the hippocampal area of many TGA patients. It has been shown that patients with DWI-positive lesions are older, and are more likely to have TIA risk factors and carotid atherosclerosis than those without [61]. Thus, at least some of the TGA cases may be due to ischemic lesions affecting the hippocampal area.

Although depression is commonly observed in survivors of stroke or TIA, it has not been considered a presenting symptom of TIA. However, pathological laughing or crying may herald major strokes, a phenomenon described by Féré in 1903 as 'fou rire prodromique' (prodrome of crazy laughter). Coelho and Ferro [62] reviewed 18 published cases of fou rire prodromique and found that fou rire can last anywhere from a few seconds to several hours. The other neurological deficits usually appeared immediately after the fou rire, but there were cases where their appearance was delayed for days or even months. Therefore, transient laughing or crying may be considered a TIA symptom in these patients.

Transient Ischemic Attack Mimics

A variety of diseases mimic TIA. Previous studies have shown that, of suspected TIAs, 18–31% are finally diagnosed as TIA mimics [22, 63, 64]. Epileptic seizures are the most important diagnosis, and other mimics include migraine, psychoneurosis, infection, toxic-metabolic diseases, syncope, TGA, vestibular disorders, spinal cord diseases, and peripheral nerve lesions. Unilateral paresis and speech disturbances are symptoms that increase the odds for TIA, whereas non-focal symptoms such as memory loss, decreased consciousness and headache are more suggestive of TIA mimics. The presence or history of cardiovascular diseases, vascular risk factors, clear neurological signs, and abnormal vascular imaging findings are closely associated with TIA, whereas abnormal signs in other (non-cerebral) organs increase the odds for TIA mimics. Therefore, careful history taking, examination of the nervous as well as other organ systems, and appropriate diagnostic tests are required for proper diagnosis.

It should be remembered that transient, and even repeated, neurological symptoms are occasionally seen in patients with non-ischemic cerebral lesions such as tumor, hemorrhages (intracerebral, subarachnoid and subdural), venous infarction, and pachymeningitis, especially when the pathology is located near the surface of the brain. The mechanism of the TIA-like symptoms in these patients remains unclear, but cortical irritation, spreading cortical depression or compression of neighboring blood vessels have all been suggested. A recent study reported on patients presenting with a cluster of stereotyped somatosensory TIA-like symptoms associated with focal, non-aneurysmal subarachnoid hemorrhages, which the authors suggested to be a forme fruste of amyloid angiopathy [65].

Specificity of Transient Ischemic Attack Symptoms and Outcome

Not every symptom is equally specific and sensitive for TIA. A recent study [66] investigated the Questionnaire for Verifying Stroke-Free Status (QVSS), originally designed to identify subjects who are free of symptomatic cerebrovascular disease, for its specificity and sensitivity for stroke/TIA. The questions include: (1) Have you ever had sudden painless weakness on one side of your body? (2) Have you ever had sudden numbness or a dead feeling on one side of your body? (3) Have you ever had sudden painless loss of vision in one or both eyes? (4) Have you ever suddenly lost one half of your vision? (5) Have you ever suddenly lost the ability to understand what people are saying? (6) Have you ever suddenly lost the ability to express yourself? When any of the QVSS questions were used, they showed a high sensitivity (0.82) and moderate specificity (0.62) for the detection of stroke/TIA. Regarding individual questions, the item showing the highest specificity was item 6 (aphasia), whereas item 2 (sensory disturbance) had the lowest specificity. The combinations of 5 and 6, and 1 and 6 had the highest specificity (0.99 each). Nevertheless, specific symptoms do not necessarily predict a high chance of development of stroke. For example, although the specificity of item 3 (TMB) is higher than item 1 (hemiparesis; 0.85 vs. 0.81, respectively), the chance for the occurrence of ipsilateral stroke in patients with TMB is only half that of those who present with hemispheric TIA [67].

Based on data on specificity of TIA symptoms and recent results showing that DWI brain lesions are most closely associated with unilateral limb weakness, followed by speech disturbances, an ABCD score was developed. It contains a clinical (item C) score: 2 points for unilateral limb weakness and 1 point for speech disturbances. As the longer duration of a patient's symptom is associated with a poorer outcome and positive DWI lesions, symptom duration was included as item D: 2 points for duration of ≥60 min and 1 point for 10–59 min [2]. Additional components include age (1 point for ≥60 years) and high blood pressure (1 point for systolic >140 mm Hg and/or diastolic ≥90 mm Hg pressure) [2]. According to Rothwell et al. [2], the ABCD score can predict the 7-day risk of stroke. Interestingly, unilateral limb weakness and speech difficulties were the symptoms most associated with an early visit to the emergency department as opposed to other symptoms such as imbalance, dizziness or confusion [68]. It has also been shown that fluctuating or unstable TIA symptoms are significantly more likely to be associated with subsequent strokes than stable symptoms [69].

However, predicting patients' outcome with the TIA symptoms alone is far from satisfactory. Recent imaging developments, such as DWI, perfusion imaging, and especially vascular imaging, have greatly enhanced our ability to predict the outcome of TIA patients [25]. This issue will be discussed in more detail in other chapters.

Recognition of Transient Ischemic Attack Symptoms

Early recognition of TIA/stroke symptoms and appropriate management to prevent further cerebrovascular events is an important issue. There have been reports that misrecognition or neglect of stroke/TIA symptoms is not uncommon in the general population. Howard et al. [70] investigated stroke/TIA symptoms in 18,462 participants who reported no stroke or TIA. The prevalence of stroke symptoms was 5.8% for sudden painless hemibody weakness, 8.5% for sudden hemibody numbness, 4.6% for sudden painless loss of vision, 3.1% for sudden hemifield visual loss, 2.7% for sudden inability to understand speech, and 3.8% for sudden inability of linguistic expression. The prevalence of one or more symptoms was 17.8%. Interestingly, symptoms were more prevalent in African-American than in Caucasian participants and in those with a lower income, a lower educational level, and a fair-to-poor perceived health status. The patients were followed for an average duration of 4.4 years, and it was found that the presence of stroke symptoms was related to stroke risk: for each stroke symptom reported, the risk of stroke increased by 21% [71].

It has also been suggested that there is a difference in recognized TIA symptoms between genders. Although TIA symptoms are not basically different between men and women, several studies have suggested that women more often present with nontraditional symptoms, such as headache, mental changes, and other nonspecific symptoms, than men [72]. Although the difference is minor, this may be related to the fact that women tend to receive slightly delayed medical attention as compared to men.

The recognition of TIA symptoms may be different between physicians, in particular between neurologists and non-neurologists. As shown in table 1, there seems to be no major differences in the assessed prevalence of major symptoms such as motor, speech and sensory disturbances between general physicians and neurologists. However, compared with neurologists, general physicians considered 'confusion' and 'unexplained fall' more often compatible with TIA and 'lower facial palsy' and 'monocular blindness' less often compatible with TIA, suggesting that the TIA concept may be understood differently. There has been suggestion that if not referred to a neurologist, one third to one half of patients labeled with a diagnosis of TIA may be inappropriately managed [73].

Misrecognition of TIA symptoms seems to be particularly more common in posterior circulation TIAs; transient isolated brainstem symptoms (e.g. isolated vertigo, dysarthria, diplopia) are not consistently classified as TIAs and easily overlooked. Recently, Paul et al. [47] reported that these symptoms preceded a vertebrobasilar stroke in 45 of 275 patients. Of all these vertebrobasilar TIA symptoms, only 8% fulfilled the National Institute of Neurological Disorders and Stroke criteria for TIA. About 22% of patients with isolated brainstem symptoms sought medical attention before the stroke, and a vascular cause was suspected by their physician in only one of these cases.

References

1 Johnston SC, Gress DR, Browner WS, Sidney S: Short-term prognosis after emergency department diagnosis of TIA. JAMA 2000;284:2901–2906.
2 Rothwell PM, Giles MF, Flossmann E, Lovelock CE, Redgrave JN, Warlow CP, Mehta Z: A simple score (ABCD) to identify individuals at high early risk of stroke after transient ischaemic attack. Lancet 2005; 366:29–36.
3 Johnston SC, Rothwell PM, Nguyen-Huynh MN, Giles MF, Elkins JS, Bernstein AL, Sidney S: Validation and refinement of scores to predict very early stroke risk after transient ischaemic attack. Lancet 2007;369:283–292.
4 Bray JE, Coughlan K, Bladin C: Can the ABCD score be dichotomised to identify high-risk patients with transient ischaemic attack in the emergency department? Emerg Med J 2007;24:92–95.
5 Calvet D, Touze E, Oppenheim C, Turc G, Meder JF, Mas JL: DWI lesions and TIA etiology improve the prediction of stroke after TIA. Stroke 2009;40:187–192.
6 Perry JJ, Sharma M, Sivilotti ML, Sutherland J, Symington C, Worster A, Emond M, Stotts G, Jin AY, Oczkowski WJ, Sahlas DJ, Murray HE, MacKey A, Verreault S, Wells GA, Stiell IG: Prospective validation of the ABCD2 score for patients in the emergency department with transient ischemic attack. CMAJ 2011;183:1137–1145.
7 Al-Khaled M, Matthis C, Munte TF, Eggers J: The incidence and clinical predictors of acute infarction in patients with transient ischemic attack using MRI including DWI. Neuroradiology 2013;55:157–163.
8 Cucchiara BL, Messe SR, Taylor RA, Pacelli J, Maus D, Shah Q, Kasner SE: Is the ABCD score useful for risk stratification of patients with acute transient ischemic attack? Stroke 2006;37:1710–1714.
9 Tsivgoulis G, Spengos K, Manta P, Karandreas N, Zambelis T, Zakopoulos N, Vassilopoulos D: Validation of the ABCD score in identifying individuals at high early risk of stroke after a transient ischemic attack: a hospital-based case series study. Stroke 2006; 37:2892–2897.
10 Lavallee PC, Meseguer E, Abboud H, Cabrejo L, Olivot JM, Simon O, Mazighi M, Nifle C, Niclot P, Lapergue B, Klein IF, Brochet E, Steg PG, Leseche G, Labreuche J, Touboul PJ, Amarenco P: A transient ischaemic attack clinic with round-the-clock access (SOS-TIA): feasibility and effects. Lancet Neurol 2007; 6:953–960.
11 Purroy F, Montaner J, Molina CA, Delgado P, Ribo M, Alvarez-Sabin J: Patterns and predictors of early risk of recurrence after transient ischemic attack with respect to etiologic subtypes. Stroke 2007;38: 3225–3229.
12 Park KY, Youn YC, Chung CS, Lee KH, Kim GM, Chung PW, Moon HS, Kim YB: Large-artery stenosis predicts subsequent vascular events in patients with transient ischemic attack. J Clin Neurol 2007;3: 169–174.
13 Sciolla R, Melis F: Rapid identification of high-risk transient ischemic attacks: prospective validation of the ABCD score. Stroke 2008;39:297–302.
14 Coutts SB, Eliasziw M, Hill MD, Scott JN, Subramaniam S, Buchan AM, Demchuk AM: An improved scoring system for identifying patients at high early risk of stroke and functional impairment after an acute transient ischemic attack or minor stroke. Int J Stroke 2008;3:3–10.
15 Amarenco P, Labreuche J, Lavallee PC, Meseguer E, Cabrejo L, Slaoui T, Guidoux C, Olivot JM, Abboud H, Lapergue B, Klein IF, Mazighi M, Touboul PJ: Does ABCD2 score below 4 allow more time to evaluate patients with a transient ischemic attack? Stroke 2009;40:3091–3095.
16 Ay H, Arsava EM, Johnston SC, Vangel M, Schwamm LH, Furie KL, Koroshetz WJ, Sorensen AG: Clinical- and imaging-based prediction of stroke risk after transient ischemic attack: the CIP model. Stroke 2009;40:181–186.
17 Sheehan OC, Merwick A, Kelly LA, Hannon N, Marnane M, Kyne L, McCormack PM, Duggan J, Moore A, Moroney J, Daly L, Harris D, Horgan G, Kelly PJ: Diagnostic usefulness of the ABCD2 score to distinguish transient ischemic attack and minor ischemic stroke from noncerebrovascular events: The North Dublin TIA study. Stroke 2009;40:3449–3454.

18 Tsivgoulis G, Stamboulis E, Sharma VK, Heliopoulos I, Voumvourakis K, Teoh HL, Patousi A, Andrikopoulou A, Lim EL, Stilou L, Sim TB, Chan BP, Stefanis L, Vadikolias K, Piperidou C: Multicenter external validation of the ABCD2 score in triaging TIA patients. Neurology 2010;74:1351–1357.
19 Nakajima M, Hirano T, Naritomi H, Minematsu K: Symptom progression or fluctuation in transient ischemic attack patients predicts subsequent stroke. Cerebrovasc Dis 2010;29:221–227.
20 Meng X, Wang Y, Liu L, Pu Y, Zhao X, Wang C: Validation of the ABCD(2)-I score to predict stroke risk after transient ischemic attack. Neurol Res 2011;33:482–486.
21 von Weitzel-Mudersbach P, Johnsen SP, Andersen G: Low risk of vascular events following urgent treatment of transient ischaemic attack: The Aarhus TIA Study. Eur J Neurol 2011;18:1285–1290.
22 Amort M, Fluri F, Schafer J, Weisskopf F, Katan M, Burow A, Bucher HC, Bonati LH, Lyrer PA, Engelter ST: Transient ischemic attack versus transient ischemic attack mimics: frequency, clinical characteristics and outcome. Cerebrovasc Dis 2011;32:57–64.
23 Cancelli I, Janes F, Gigli GL, Perelli A, Zanchettin B, Canal G, D'Anna L, Russo V, Barbone F, Valente M: Incidence of transient ischemic attack and early stroke risk: validation of the ABCD2 score in an Italian population-based study. Stroke 2011;42:2751–2757.
24 Poisson SN, Nguyen-Huynh MN, Johnston SC, Furie KL, Lev MH, Smith WS: Intracranial large vessel occlusion as a predictor of decline in functional status after transient ischemic attack. Stroke 2011;42:44–47.
25 Purroy F, Jimenez Caballero PE, Gorospe A, Torres MJ, Alvarez-Sabin J, Santamarina E, Martinez-Sanchez P, Canovas D, Freijo MM, Egido JA, Giron JM, Ramirez-Moreno JM, Alonso A, Rodriguez-Campello A, Casado I, Delgado-Medeiros R, Marti-Fabregas J, Fuentes B, Silva Y, Quesada H, Cardona P, Morales A, de la Ossa N, Garcia-Pastor A, Arenillas JF, Segura T, Jimenez C, Masjuan J: Prediction of early stroke recurrence in transient ischemic attack patients from the PROMAPA study: a comparison of prognostic risk scores. Cerebrovasc Dis 2012;33:182–189.
26 Coutts SB, Modi J, Patel SK, Demchuk AM, Goyal M, Hill MD: CT/CT angiography and MRI findings predict recurrent stroke after transient ischemic attack and minor stroke: results of the prospective CATCH study. Stroke 2012;43:1013–1017.
27 Dolatabadi A, Meisami A, Hatamabadi H, Mansori B, Shahrami A, Amini A, Jamali K: Improving the prediction of stroke or death after transient ischemic attack (TIA) by adding diffusion-weighted imaging lesions and TIA etiology to the ABCD2 score. J Stroke Cerebrovasc Dis 2012, E-pub ahead of print.
28 Hoshino T, Nagao T, Mizuno S, Shimizu S, Uchiyama S: Cardioembolic stroke is frequent in late recurrence after transient ischemic attack. J Stroke Cerebrovasc Dis 2012, E-pub ahead of print.
29 Donnan GA, O'Malley HM, Quang L, Hurley S, Bladin PF: The capsular warning syndrome: pathogenesis and clinical features. Neurology 1993;43:957–962.
30 Farrar J, Donnan GA: Capsular warning syndrome preceding pontine infarction. Stroke 1993;24:762.
31 Paul NL, Simoni M, Chandratheva A, Rothwell PM: Population-based study of capsular warning syndrome and prognosis after early recurrent TIA. Neurology 2012;79:1356–1362.
32 Fisher CM: Pure sensory stroke and allied conditions. Stroke 1982;13:434–447.
33 Kim JS: Pure or predominantly sensory transient ischemic attacks associated with posterior cerebral artery stenosis. Cerebrovasc Dis 2002;14:136–138.
34 Martin R, Bogousslavsky J, Regli F: Pure sensory stroke heralding large hemispheric infarction. Schweiz Arch Neurol Psychiatr 1992;143:339–342.
35 Kim JS: Bilateral perioral sensory symptom after unilateral stroke: does it have a localizing value? J Neurol Sci 1996;140:123–128.
36 Kimura K, Minematsu K, Wada K, Yonemura K, Nakajima M: Clinical characteristics in transient ischemic attack patients with atrial fibrillation. Intern Med 2003;42:255–258.
37 Fisher CM: 'Transient monocular blindness' versus 'amaurosis fugax'. Neurology 1989;39:1622–1624.
38 Fisher M: Transient monocular blindness associated with hemiplegia. AMA Arch Ophthalmol 1952;47: 167–203.
39 Savino PJ, Glaser JS, Cassady J: Retinal stroke. Is the patient at risk? Arch Ophthalmol 1977;95:1185–1189.
40 Howard RS, Russell RW: Prognosis of patients with retinal embolism. J Neurol Neurosurg Psychiatry 1987;50:1142–1147.
41 Furlan AJ, Whisnant JP, Kearns TP: Unilateral visual loss in bright light. An unusual symptom of carotid artery occlusive disease. Arch Neurol 1979;36: 675–676.
42 Wiebers DO, Swanson JW, Cascino TL, Whisnant JP: Bilateral loss of vision in bright light. Stroke 1989; 20:554–558.
43 Winterkorn JM, Kupersmith MJ, Wirtschafter JD, Forman S: Brief report: treatment of vasospastic amaurosis fugax with calcium-channel blockers. N Engl J Med 1993;329:396–398.
44 Falke P, Abela BM Jr, Krakau CE, Lilja B, Lindgarde F, Maly P, Stavenow L: High frequency of asymptomatic visual field defects in subjects with transient ischaemic attacks or minor strokes. J Intern Med 1991;229:521–525.
45 Krasnianski M, Bau V, Neudecker S, Lindner A, Zierz S: Isolated bilateral blindness as the sole manifestation of transient ischaemic attacks. Acta Ophthalmol Scand 2006;84:415–418.
46 Hoshino T, Nagao T, Mizuno S, Shimizu S, Uchiyama S: Transient neurological attack before vertebrobasilar stroke. J Neurol Sci 2013;325:39–42.

47 Paul NL, Simoni M, Rothwell PM: Transient isolated brainstem symptoms preceding posterior circulation stroke: a population-based study. Lancet Neurol 2013;12:65–71.
48 Kerber KA, Brown DL, Lisabeth LD, Smith MA, Morgenstern LB: Stroke among patients with dizziness, vertigo, and imbalance in the emergency department: a population-based study. Stroke 2006;37:2484–2487.
49 Kapoor WN, Karpf M, Wieand S, Peterson JR, Levey GS: A prospective evaluation and follow-up of patients with syncope. N Engl J Med 1983;309:197–204.
50 Eagle KA, Black HR, Cook EF, Goldman L: Evaluation of prognostic classifications for patients with syncope. Am J Med 1985;79:455–460.
51 Davidson E, Rotenbeg Z, Fuchs J, Weinberger I, Agmon J: Transient ischemic attack-related syncope. Clin Cardiol 1991;14:141–144.
52 Bianchi A, Baldini E, Suppa M, Rosa A, Coppola A, Cavicchi F, Contu E, Petroni C, Strano S, Scarpellini MG: The syncope in emergency department: usual management vs guidelines (in Italian). Clin Ter 2011;162:e73–e77.
53 Loeb C, Gandolfo C, Dall'Agata D: Headache in transient ischemic attacks (TIA). Cephalalgia 1985; 5(suppl 2):17–19.
54 Andre C, Neves FF, Vincent MB: Headache in transient ischaemic attacks. Funct Neurol 1996;11:195–200.
55 Andre C, Vincent MB: On the pathogenesis of headache following TIA. Arq Neuropsiquiatr 1997;55: 167–173.
56 Baquis GD, Pessin MS, Scott RM: Limb shaking – a carotid TIA. Stroke 1985;16:444–448.
57 Jiang WJ, Gao F, Du B, Srivastava T, Wang YJ: Limb-shaking transient ischemic attack induced by middle cerebral artery stenosis. Cerebrovasc Dis 2006;21: 421–422.
58 Han SW, Kim SH, Kim JK, Park CH, Yun MJ, Heo JH: Hemodynamic changes in limb shaking TIA associated with anterior cerebral artery stenosis. Neurology 2004;63:1519–1521.
59 Kim JS: Asterixis after unilateral stroke: lesion location of 30 patients. Neurology 2001;56:533–536.
60 Spengos K, Tsivgoulis G, Toulas P, Vemmos K, Vassilopoulos D, Spengos M: Hyperventilation-enhanced chorea as a transient ischaemic phenomenon in a patient with moyamoya disease. Eur Neurol 2004;51:172–175.
61 Winbeck K, Etgen T, von Einsiedel HG, Rottinger M, Sander D: DWI in transient global amnesia and TIA: proposal for an ischaemic origin of TGA. J Neurol Neurosurg Psychiatry 2005;76:438–441.
62 Coelho M, Ferro JM: Fou rire prodromique. Case report and systematic review of literature. Cerebrovasc Dis 2003;16:101–104.
63 Libman RB, Wirkowski E, Alvir J, Rao TH: Conditions that mimic stroke in the emergency department. Implications for acute stroke trials. Arch Neurol 1995;52:1119–1122.
64 Hand PJ, Kwan J, Lindley RI, Dennis MS, Wardlaw JM: Distinguishing between stroke and mimic at the bedside: The brain attack study. Stroke 2006;37:769–775.
65 Izenberg A, Aviv RI, Demaerschalk BM, Dodick DW, Hopyan J, Black SE, Gladstone DJ: Crescendo transient aura attacks: a transient ischemic attack mimic caused by focal subarachnoid hemorrhage. Stroke 2009;40:3725–3729.
66 Sung VW, Johnson N, Granstaff US, Jones WJ, Meschia JF, Williams LS, Safford MM: Sensitivity and specificity of stroke symptom questions to detect stroke or transient ischemic attack. Neuroepidemiology 2011;36:100–104.
67 Benavente O, Eliasziw M, Streifler JY, Fox AJ, Barnett HJ, Meldrum H: Prognosis after transient monocular blindness associated with carotid-artery stenosis. N Engl J Med 2001;345:1084–1090.
68 Gargano JW, Wehner S, Reeves MJ: Presenting symptoms and onset-to-arrival time in patients with acute stroke and transient ischemic attack. J Stroke Cerebrovasc Dis 2011;20:494–502.
69 Chatzikonstantinou A, Willmann O, Jager T, Szabo K, Hennerici MG: Transient ischemic attack patients with fluctuations are at highest risk for early stroke. Cerebrovasc Dis 2009;27:594–598.
70 Howard VJ, McClure LA, Meschia JF, Pulley L, Orr SC, Friday GH: High prevalence of stroke symptoms among persons without a diagnosis of stroke or transient ischemic attack in a general population: the reasons for geographic and racial differences in stroke (REGARDS) study. Arch Intern Med 2006;166: 1952–1958.
71 Kleindorfer D, Judd S, Howard VJ, McClure L, Safford MM, Cushman M, Rhodes D, Howard G: Self-reported stroke symptoms without a prior diagnosis of stroke or transient ischemic attack: a powerful new risk factor for stroke. Stroke 2011;42:3122–3126.
72 Lisabeth LD, Brown DL, Hughes R, Majersik JJ, Morgenstern LB: Acute stroke symptoms: comparing women and men. Stroke 2009;40:2031–2036.
73 Ferro JM, Falcao I, Rodrigues G, Canhao P, Melo TP, Oliveira V, Pinto AN, Crespo M, Salgado AV: Diagnosis of transient ischemic attack by the nonneurologist. A validation study. Stroke 1996;27:2225–2229.

Jong S. Kim, MD, PhD
University of Ulsan, Stroke Center, Asan Medical Center
388-1 Pungnap-dong, Songpa-gu
Seoul 138-736 (South Korea)
E-Mail jongskim@amc.seoul.kr

Uchiyama S, Amarenco P, Minematsu K, Wong KSL (eds): TIA as Acute Cerebrovascular Syndrome.
Front Neurol Neurosci. Basel, Karger, 2014, vol 33, pp 103–114 (DOI: 10.1159/000351911)

Guidelines for Management of Patients with Transient Ischemic Attack

Toshiyuki Uehara · Kazuo Minematsu
National Cerebral and Cardiovascular Center, Osaka, Japan

Abstract

A transient ischemic attack (TIA) is a medical emergency that is associated with a high risk of early ischemic stroke and other vascular events. Several evidence-based guidelines have been published to provide recommendations for the evaluation and treatment of patients with TIA. These guidelines underline the need for the urgent referral of patients with TIA so that they can access expert evaluation and immediate treatment. The distinction between TIA and ischemic stroke has recently become less important because these two conditions share pathophysiological mechanisms and many of the preventive approaches are applicable to both. Therefore, current guidelines are often described without a distinction between TIA and ischemic stroke. However, the applicability of recommendations for applying treatment for ischemic stroke to TIA has not been proven. Further studies are required to determine the effects of urgent intervention or treatment early after TIA.

A transient ischemic attack (TIA) is a medical emergency that is associated with a high risk of early ischemic stroke and other vascular events. Among patients with TIA, 10–15% develop stroke within 90 days, with about half occurring within 48 h [1–4]. Urgent assessment and management of patients in a dedicated TIA clinic has decreased the 90-day stroke risk by almost 80% [5, 6]. Patients with TIA are also at high risk of cardiovascular events [1]. A previous study found that 2.6% of patients were hospitalized for major cardiovascular events including myocardial infarction, unstable angina, or ventricular arrhythmia within 90 days of TIA [7]. These findings underline the need for the urgent referral of patients with TIA so that they can access expert evaluations and immediate treatment. Several evidenced-based guidelines have provided recommendations for the evaluation and treatment of patients with TIA [8–24].

T.U. and K.M. contributed equally to this chapter.

The classical definition of TIA is the presence of focal neurological symptoms ascribable to a vascular etiology lasting <24 h irrespective of imaging findings [25]. The advent of brain imaging techniques has led to the understanding that up to one third of patients with symptoms lasting <24 h actually has an infarction [1]. This has led to a new tissue-based definition of TIA, that is 'a transient episode of neurological dysfunction caused by focal brain, spinal cord or retinal ischemia, without acute infarction' [1], which is different from the traditional time-based definition. According to this definition, the diagnostic certainty of TIA would depend on the extent of evaluations that a patient undergoes. A brain imaging procedure is prerequisite for concluding a diagnosis of TIA or ischemic stroke.

In contrast, the distinction between TIA and ischemic stroke has become less important because these two conditions share the same pathophysiological mechanisms, and many of the preventive approaches are applicable to both [1]. Acute ischemic stroke and TIA in the acute setting are considered to span the same spectrum, and a new clinical concept termed acute cerebrovascular syndrome has been proposed [26]. Current guidelines are usually presented without a distinction between TIA and ischemic stroke.

We present representative guidelines for the management of patients with TIA [8–24].

Representative Guidelines for the Management of Transient Ischemic Attack

A panel of the American Heart Association (AHA) Stroke Council published 'Guidelines for the management of transient ischemic attacks' in 1994 and a supplement in 1999, and both were separate from the guidelines for the management of stroke [8, 9]. The AHA/American Stroke Association (ASA) issued a scientific statement for the definition and evaluation of TIA in 2009 [1]. The National Stroke Association (NSA) published guidelines for the management of TIA in 2006, and recommendations for systems of care for TIA in 2011 [10, 11]. Guidelines for the assessment and management of people with recent TIA were published in New Zealand in 2008 [12]. A chapter for TIA management was newly added in the second edition of the guidelines for management of stroke in Japan in 2009. The English version of the Japanese guidelines was published recently [13]. A separate chapter for the management of TIA was similarly described in guidelines for management of stroke in the UK [14, 15] and Australia [16]. The AHA/ASA published a scientific statement for 'Coronary risk evaluation in patients with transient ischemic attack and ischemic stroke' in 2003 [17], and 'Guidelines for the prevention of stroke in patients with stroke or transient ischemic attack' in 2006, 2008 and 2011 [18–20], without a distinction between stroke and TIA. 'Guidelines for management of ischaemic stroke and transient ischaemic attack' published in 2008 by the European Stroke Organization (ESO) [21] is an update of the European Stroke Initiative (EUSI) Recommendations for Stroke Management published in 2000. The American College of Chest Physicians evidence-based clinical practice guidelines for antithrombotic and thrombolytic therapy for ischemic stroke [22], a Science Advisory of AHA/ASA for oral antithrombotic agents for the prevention of stroke in nonvalvular atrial fibrillation (AF) [23], and an update of the 2010 ESC guidelines for the management of AF [24] covered both ischemic stroke and TIA.

Risk Stratification for Referral to a Specialized Hospital

Patients with suspected TIA require a differential diagnosis from TIA mimics, an assessment of vascular risk factors, and investigations to determine the potential causes of TIA. Magnetic resonance imaging (MRI), including diffusion-weighted imaging (DWI) sequences should be the preferred diagnostic test for patients with suspected TIA. An additional diagnostic workup, including vessel imaging, cardiac evaluation and laboratory testing, should be completed as soon as possible, preferably within hours or a day or two.

To determine the short-term risk of stroke facing the individual patient is important. Patients at high risk of subsequent stroke would benefit more by urgent referral to a specialized stroke center, timely identification of the underlying etiology, and preventive measures such as antiplatelet agents, anticoagulants, and carotid endarterectomy (CEA). Admitting high-risk patients to specialized stroke centers might also provide opportunities to administer acute timely treatments in the event of a subsequent stroke [27].

Simple stratification scores are used to estimate the individual risk for patients with TIA. The most popular tool is the $ABCD^2$ score [28]. The $ABCD^2$ score is recommended to identify patients at high risk of stroke in several guidelines [1, 10, 12, 14–16], and it can be used in primary care to select patients for referral to specialized stroke centers. The presence of ischemic lesions on DWI and TIA etiology, such as large artery atherosclerosis and AF, could improve stroke risk prediction after TIA. However, clinical plus imaging scores, such as the $ABCD^2$-I [29], require additional estimations, and are more difficult to apply. Although these scores could be used in specialized stroke centers to individualize TIA management, they cannot be applied in primary care.

Initial Management and Estimations

Guidelines of the ESO [21]

The ESO guidelines recommend that patients with suspected TIA be referred without delay to a TIA clinic or to a medical center with a stroke unit that can provide expert evaluation and immediate treatment. An immediate diagnostic workup, including urgent vascular imaging (ultrasound, CT or MR angiography), is recommended for patients with TIA, minor stroke or early spontaneous recovery.

National Clinical Guidelines of the National Institute for Clinical Excellence [14]
The National Institute for Clinical Excellence (NICE) guidelines recommend that all patients with TIA should be given immediate antiplatelet therapy with 300 mg/day of aspirin and then referred for urgent specialist assessment. The NICE guidelines recommend that individuals with suspected TIA and at high risk for stroke (for example, $ABCD^2$ score ≥4 or with crescendo TIA) in whom the vascular territory or pathology is uncertain should undergo urgent (within 24 h) brain imaging studies (preferably DWI). Those with suspected TIA at low risk for stroke (for example, $ABCD^2$ <4) in whom the vascular territory or pathology is uncertain should undergo brain imaging studies (preferably DWI) within 7 days. Individuals with suspected TIA who require brain imaging due to uncertain vascular territory or pathology should undergo DWI except where contraindicated, in which case CT scanning should be used (fig. 1a).

National Stroke Strategy of the Department of Health (UK) in 2007 [15]
This strategy recommends immediate referral for appropriately urgent specialist assessment and an assessment of all patients presenting with recent TIA or minor stroke. All higher-risk patients with TIA and minor stroke (e.g. $ABCD^2$ score ≥4) need to be assessed by a specialist and treated within 24 h. Immediate hospital admission might be justified for those at highest risk. High-risk patients who are not considered to require immediate hospital admission have better outcomes if they are assessed, investigated and treated within 24 h of referral. Lower-risk patients with TIA or minor stroke are best assessed within 7 days of the event. Non-urgent referral for TIA or minor stroke is appropriate only for very low-risk patients, such as those presenting with events that occurred several weeks or months previously (fig. 1b).

Clinical Guidelines by National Stroke Foundation (Australia) in 2010 [16]
These guidelines recommend that all patients with suspected TIA should have a full assessment including a detailed history and clinical, prognostic (e.g. $ABCD^2$ score) and investigative tests (e.g. blood tests, brain and carotid imaging and electrocardiography, ECG) at the initial point of healthcare contact, regardless of whether it is in primary or secondary care. Patients identified as being at high risk (e.g. $ABCD^2$ score ≥4 and/or any one of AF, carotid territory symptoms or crescendo TIA) should undergo urgent brain assessment preferably MRI with DWI and carotid imaging within 24 h. In settings with limited access to such modalities, patients should be referred within 24 h to the nearest center where such assessments can be quickly conducted. Patients classified as low risk (e.g. $ABCD^2$ score <4 without AF or carotid territory symptoms or who present more than one week after the last symptoms) should be assessed by brain and carotid imaging as soon as possible, preferably within 48 h (fig. 1c).

Guidelines of Stroke Foundation of New Zealand [12]
The New Zealand guidelines recommend an assessment of stroke risk for all patients with suspected TIA using the $ABCD^2$ tool at the initial point of health care contact

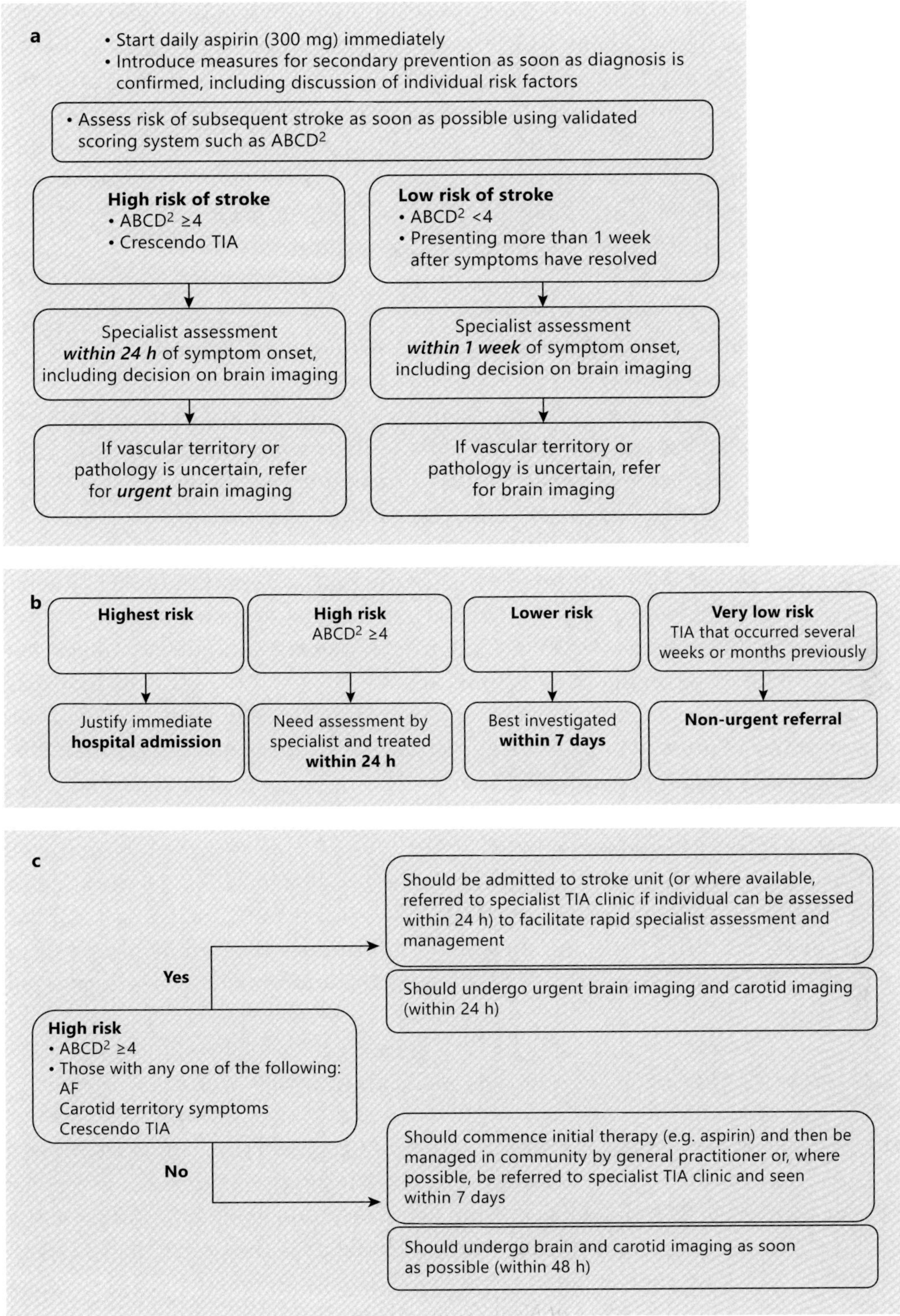

Fig. 1. Algorithms for initial management and estimations. **a** Guidelines of NICE [14]. **b** National Stroke Strategy (UK) [15]. **c** Guidelines of National Stroke Foundation (Australia) [16].

regardless of whether in primary or secondary care. High risk is indicated by any of the following: presence of symptoms at first contact; $ABCD^2$ score ≥4; crescendo TIAs, AF or already receiving anticoagulation therapy. Low risk is indicated by any of the following: $ABCD^2$ score <4 and late presentation (one week after symptoms appear).

Guidelines in Japan [13]

The Japanese guidelines recommend evaluating patients with suspected TIA to identify the onset mechanism and initiating treatment as soon as possible after TIA onset to prevent subsequent cerebral infarction.

Scientific Statement for Definition and Evaluation of Transient Ischemic Attack Published by AHA/ASA in 2009 [1]

This statement recommends evaluating patients with suspected TIA as soon as possible after an event. Patients with TIA should preferably undergo neuroimaging evaluation within 24 h of symptom onset, and MRI, including DWI, is the preferred brain diagnostic imaging modality. If MRI is not available, head CT should be performed. The cervicocephalic vessels should be imaged noninvasively as part of the routine evaluation of patients with suspected TIAs. Noninvasive assessment of the intracranial vasculature reliably excludes intracranial stenosis, and the likelihood of intracranial steno-occlusive disease that would alter management can be determined. Patients should be assessed by ECG as soon as possible after TIA. Prolonged cardiac monitoring (inpatient telemetry or Holter monitoring) is useful for patients with an unclear origin after initial brain imaging and electrocardiography. At least transthoracic echocardiography is reasonable when evaluating patients with suspected TIAs, especially when no cause has been identified by other elements of the workup. Transesophageal echocardiography is useful in identifying patent foramen ovale, aortic arch atherosclerosis and valvular disease, and is reasonable when identification of these conditions will alter management. Routine blood tests, including complete blood count, chemistry panel, prothrombin time and partial thromboplastin time, and fasting lipid panel, are reasonable in the evaluation of patients with suspected TIAs.

National Stroke Association Guidelines for the Management of Transient Ischemic Attacks [10]

These guidelines recommend establishing specialized clinics for the rapid assessment of TIA within 24–48 h of diagnosis. Physicians and institutions that provide care for patients with recent TIA should have same-day access to imaging modalities such as CT/CTA, MR/MR angiography and ultrasound for patients who need it. Patients with suspected TIA who are not admitted to hospital should have rapid (within 12 h) access for urgent assessment and investigation by CT or MRI brain scanning, ECG and carotid Doppler ultrasonography. Patients should be initially assessed within 24–48 h if they are not already assessed by cross-sectional imaging, ECG, or carotid ultrasound in the emergency department. If they have been performed and the findings are negative, up to 7 days might be appropriate. Patients with a TIA within the past 2 weeks but who were not hospitalized, should undergo prompt (within 24–48 h) assessments by means of carotid Doppler ultrasonography for TIA consistent with carotid territory, blood work and cardiac evaluation using ECG, rhythm strip, and echocardiography to determine the mechanism of ischemia and subsequent preventive therapy.

Hospital Admission

Ideally, all patients with suspected TIA should be immediately hospitalized to ensure rapid diagnostic evaluation and acute stroke therapies. However, admitting all patients with suspected TIA would probably be problematic, as hospital resources (staff and beds) would become insufficient and costs would soar. Neither 100% hospitalization nor 100% outpatient evaluation of patients with TIA is ideal. For acute hospitalization after suspected TIA, risk stratification in the emergency room might help triage patients (high risk) for hospitalization and outpatient (low risk) management [30]. The $ABCD^2$ score can function in this role. In addition, the presence of ischemic lesions on DWI and an apparent TIA etiology, such as large artery atherosclerosis and AF, could improve stroke risk predictions after TIA.

The NSA evidence-based guidelines for TIA management [10] state that hospitalization should be considered for patients with a first TIA within the past 24–48 h to facilitate the possible early deployment of lytic therapy and other medical management strategies if symptoms recur and to expedite the institution of definitive secondary prevention. Additionally, timely hospital referral for a recent TIA (within one week) is always advisable, and hospital admission is generally recommended in the case of crescendo TIAs or duration of symptoms for more than 1 h, symptomatic internal carotid artery stenosis >50% in diameter, a known cardiac source of embolus such as AF, a known hypercoagulable state, or an appropriate combination of the California or ABCD scores.

The scientific statement of AHA/ASA [1] recommends admitting patients with TIA to hospital if they present within 72 h of the event and if any of the following criteria are present: $ABCD^2$ score of ≥3, $ABCD^2$ score 0–2 and uncertainty that diagnostic workup can be completed within 2 days as an outpatient, or $ABCD^2$ score 0–2 and other evidence indicating that focal ischemia caused the event.

The Clinical Guidelines for Acute Stroke Management published by the National Stroke Foundation [16] describe that all patients with suspected TIA presenting to a general practitioner or emergency department should be rapidly assessed. Those identified as high risk ($ABCD^2$ score ≥4 and/or those with any of AF, carotid territory symptoms or crescendo TIA) should be admitted to a stroke unit (or where available, referred to a specialist TIA clinic if they can be assessed within 24 h) to facilitate rapid specialist assessment and management. Those identified as low risk ($ABCD^2$ score <4 and without AF or carotid territory symptoms or crescendo TIA) should start initial therapy (e.g. aspirin) and then be managed in the community setting by a general practitioner or private specialist or, where possible, be referred to a specialist TIA clinic and seen within 7 days (fig. 1c).

Treatment

All patients with TIA are at risk of subsequent stroke and cardiovascular events including myocardial infarction and death. Several interventions that have proven effective in preventing these events are covered by international guidelines and include anticoagulation for cardioembolic TIA, antiplatelet therapy for non-cardioembolic TIA, CEA for >50% symptomatic carotid stenosis, blood pressure (BP)-lowering drugs, statins, improved glycemic control, dietary modification, exercise and smoking cessation [12]. Patients with suspected TIA should be evaluated to determine etiology and be treated to prevent subsequent stroke as soon as possible after TIA onset.

Antiplatelet Therapy

The NICE [14] and Stroke Foundation of New Zealand [12] guidelines recommended starting antiplatelet therapy immediately for all individuals with suspected TIA until brain imaging results are available. Primary intracerebral hemorrhage (ICH) is a rare cause of TIA, and 99% of strokes after TIA are due to cerebral infarction, and no clear evidence indicates that the inadvertent administration of aspirin to patients with ICH before imaging is harmful [12]. Japanese guidelines recommend administering 160–300 mg/day of aspirin for patients with acute TIA (within 48 h) [13]. Daily long-term antiplatelet therapy should be prescribed immediately for the secondary prevention of stroke and other vascular events in patients with non-cardioembolic TIA. Aspirin monotherapy (50–325 mg/day), aspirin (25 mg) combined with extended-release dipyridamole (200 mg) twice daily, and monotherapy with clopidogrel (75 mg) are all acceptable options for initial therapy [10, 20–22]. In addition, cilostazol (200 mg/day) is recommended by the American College of Chest Physicians Evidence-based Clinical Practice Guidelines [22]. Antiplatelet agents that can be applied in Japan comprise aspirin (75–150 mg/day), clopidogrel (75 mg), cilostazol (200 mg/day) and ticlopidine (200 mg/day) [13]. Combining aspirin with clopidogrel increases risk of hemorrhage and is not recommended for long-term secondary prevention after TIA [16, 20, 21].

Anticoagulation Therapy

Long-term oral anticoagulation with a target international normalized ratio (INR) of 2.5 (range, 2.0–3.0) is recommended for patients with TIA and emboligenic cardiac diseases such as persistent or paroxysmal valvular or nonvalvular AF [10, 12, 16, 20–23]. The Japanese guidelines recommend a target INR range of 2.0–3.0 for patients aged <70 years of age and 1.6–2.6 in those aged ≥70 years [13]. The American College of Chest Physicians Evidence-based Clinical Practice Guidelines [22] recommend oral anticoagulation therapy with dabigatran (150 mg b.i.d.) over adjusted-dose vitamin K antagonist therapy for patients with a history of ischemic stroke or TIA and AF, including paroxysmal AF. The AHA/ASA Science Advisory for oral antithrombotic agents for the prevention of stroke in nonvalvular AF recommends warfarin, dabigatran, apixaban, and rivaroxaban to prevent a first and recurrent stroke in patients with nonvalvular AF [23]. The selection of an antithrombotic agent should be individualized on the basis of risk factors, cost, tolerability, patient preference, potential for drug interactions and other clinical characteristics, including time in the INR therapeutic range if the patient has been treated with warfarin [23]. An update of the 2010 ESC guidelines for the management of AF recommends that novel oral anticoagulant drugs, including dabigatran, apixaban, and rivaroxaban, should be considered instead of adjusted-dose vitamin K antagonist [24].

Carotid Revascularization

CEA is recommended for patients with recent TIA and ipsilateral severe carotid artery stenosis (70–99%). For patients with recent TIA and ipsilateral moderate carotid stenosis (50–69%), CEA is recommended depending on patient-specific factors such as age, sex, and comorbidities. When the degree of stenosis is <50%, there is no indication for CEA. Carotid artery stenting is indicated in patients at a high risk of CEA, such as those with coronary artery disease [10, 12, 13, 16, 20, 21]. In patients with symptomatic internal carotid artery stenosis for whom CEA is a reasonable option, surgery should be performed as soon as the patient is fit for the procedure, preferably within 2 weeks of TIA (cerebral or retinal) [10, 14, 16, 20].

Treatment to Reduce the Cardiovascular Risk

All individuals with a history of TIA should be considered for treatment to reduce cardiovascular risk, and risk factors for recurrent cerebrovascular ischemic events should be appropriately treated. This includes lowering BP and blood cholesterol (with lifestyle modifications and/or drug therapy) for all patients with atherothrombotic TIA, regardless of baseline BP and cholesterol values [10]. The New Zealand guidelines recommend assessing every individual with TIA and informing them of their risk factors for stroke and adverse cardiovascular events, and of possible strategies to modify identified risk factors [12].

Blood Pressure Lowering

Reducing BP is recommended to prevent both recurrent stroke and other vascular events from arising in persons who have had an ischemic stroke or TIA and are beyond the first 24 h [20]. The absolute target BP is uncertain but a benefit has been associated with an average reduction of about 10/5 mm Hg, and normal BP levels have been defined as <120/80 mm Hg [20, 21]. After TIA that is not due to dissection or cardiogenic embolism, BP should be reduced to <140/90 or <130/80 mm Hg for diabetics, regardless of the initial level, unless the patient has symptomatic hypotension. An angiotensin-converting enzyme inhibitor alone or in combination with a diuretic, or with an angiotensin receptor blocker is useful [10, 20].

Cholesterol Lowering
Statin therapy with intensive lipid-lowering effects is recommended to reduce the risk of stroke and cardiovascular events among patients with ischemic stroke or TIA who have evidence of atherosclerosis, an LDL-C level of >100 mg/dl, and who are without known coronary heart disease [20].

Diabetes Management
Fasting blood glucose levels of <126 mg/dl (7 mmol/l) are recommended. Diet, exercise at least three times a week and oral hypoglycemic agents or insulin should be prescribed as needed to control diabetes for the long-term secondary prevention of stroke [9]. Diabetes should be managed with lifestyle modification and individualized pharmacological therapy [21].

Behavioral Changes
Cessation of smoking, maintaining an appropriate body weight, and enforced exercise are recommended to reduce the risk of recurrent TIA or stroke [10, 12–16, 20].

References

1 Easton JD, Saver JL, Albers GW, Alberts MJ, Chaturvedi S, Feldmann E, Hatsukami TS, Higashida RT, Johnston SC, Kidwell CS, Lustep HL, Miller E, Sacco RL: Definition and evaluation of transient ischemic attack: a scientific statement for healthcare professionals from the American Heart Association/American Stroke Association Stroke Council; Council on Cardio-Vascular Surgery and Anesthesia; Council on Cardiovascular Radiology and Intervention; Council on Cardiovascular Nursing; and the Interdisciplinary Council on Peripheral Vascular Disease. The American Academy of Neurology affirms the value of this statement as an educational tool for neurologists. Stroke 2009;40:2276–2293.

2 Giles MF, Rothwell PM: Risk of stroke early after transient ischaemic attack: a systematic review and meta-analysis. Lancet Neurol 2007;6:1063–1072.

3 Wu CM, McLaughlin K, Lorenzetti DL, Hill MD, Manns BJ, Ghali WA: Early risk of stroke after transient ischemic attack: a systematic review and meta-analysis. Arch Intern Med 2007;167:2417–2422.

4 Redgrave JN, Coutts SB, Schulz UG, Briley D, Rothwell PM: Systematic review of associations between the presence of acute ischemic lesions on diffusion-weighted imaging and clinical predictors of early stroke risk after transient ischemic attack. Stroke 2007;38:1482–1488.

5 Lavallee PC, Meseguer E, Abboud H, Cabrejo L, Olivot JM, Simon O, Mazighi M, Nicolt P, Lapergue B, Klein IF, Brochet E, Steg PG, Leseche G, Labreuche J, Touboul PJ, Amarenco P: A transient ischemic attack clinic with round-the-clock access (SOS-TIA): feasibility and effects. Lancet Neurol 2007;6:953–960.

6 Rothwell PM, Giles MF, Chandratheva A, Marquardt L, Geraghty O, Redgrave JN, Lovelock CE, Binney LE, Bull LM, Cuthberton FC, Welch SJ, Bosch S, Alexander FC, Silver LE, Gutnikov SA, Mehta Z: Effect of urgent treatment of transient ischaemic attack and minor stroke on early recurrent stroke (EXPRESS study): a prospective population-based sequential comparison. Lancet 2007;370:1432–1442.

7 Elkins JS, Sidney S, Gress DR, Go AS, Bernstein AL, Johnston SC: Electrocardiographic findings predict short-term cardiac morbidity after transient ischemic attack. Arch Neurol 2002;59:1437–1441.
8 Feinberg WM, Albers GW, Barnett HJ, Biller J, Caplan LR, Carter LP, Hart RG, Hobson RW II, Kronmal RA, Moore WS, Robertson JT, Adams HP Jr, Mayberg M: Guidelines for the management of transient ischemic attacks: from the Ad Hoc Committee on Guidelines for the Management of Transient Ischemic Attacks of the Stroke Council of the American Heart Association. AHA medical/scientific statement: special report. Circulation 1994;89: 2950–2965.
9 Albers GW, Hart RG, Lutsep HL, Newell DW, Sacco RL: AHA Scientific Statement. Supplement to the guidelines for the management of transient ischemic attacks: a statement from the Ad Hoc Committee on Guidelines for the Management of Transient Ischemic Attacks, Stroke Council, American Heart Association. Stroke 1999;30:2502–2511.
10 Johnston SC, Nguyen-Huynh MN, Schwarz ME, Fuller K, Williams CE, Josephson SA, Hankey GJ, Hart RG, Levine SR, Biller J, Brown RD Jr, Sacco RL, Kappelle LJ, Koudstaal PJ, Bogousslavsky J, Caplan LR, van Gijn J, Algra A, Rothwell PM, Adams HP, Albers GW: National Stroke Association guidelines for the management of transient ischemic attacks. Ann Neurol 2006;60:301–313.
11 Johnston SC, Albers GW, Gorelick PB, Cumbler E, Klingman J, Ross MA, Briggs M, Carlton J, Sloan EP, Vaince U: National Stroke Association recommendations for systems of care for transient ischemic attack. Ann Neurol 2011;69:872–877.
12 New Zealand guideline for the assessment and management of people with recent transient ischemic attack (TIA). Wellington, Stroke Foundation of New Zealand, 2008. http://www.stroke.org.nz/resources/TIA_GuidelineForweb.pdf.
13 Shinohara Y, Yanagihara T, Abe K, Yoshimine T, Fujinaka T, Chuma T, Ochi F, Nagayama M, Ogawa A, Suzuki N, Katayama Y, Kimura A, Minematsu K: Cerebral infarction/transient ischemic attack (TIA). Japanese Guidelines for the Management of Stroke 2009. J Stroke Cerebrovasc Dis 2011;45:S31–S73.
14 National Collaborating Centre for Chronic Conditions (UK): Stroke: National clinical guideline for diagnosis and initial management of acute stroke and transient ischaemic attack (TIA). National Institute for Health and Clinical Excellence: Guidance. London, Royal College of Physicians (UK), 2008.
15 Stroke Team, Vascular Programme, Department of Health. National Stroke Strategy. London, Department of Health, 2007. http://www.dh.gov.uk/en/Publicationsandstatistics/Publications/PublicationsPolicyAndGuidance/DH_081062.
16 Clinical Guidelines for Stroke Management 2010. Melbourne, National Stroke Foundation, 2010. http://strokefoundation.com.au/site/media/clinical_guidelines_stroke_managment_2010_interactive.pdf.
17 Adams RJ, Chimowitz MI, Alpert JS, Awad IA, Cerqueria MD, Fayad P, Taubert KA: Coronary risk evaluation in patients with transient ischemic attack and ischemic stroke: a scientific statement for healthcare professionals from the Stroke Council and the Council on Clinical Cardiology of the American Heart Association/American Stroke Association. Stroke 2003;34:2310–2322.
18 Sacco RL, Adams R, Albers G, Alberts MJ, Benavente O, Furie K, Goldstein LB, Gorelick P, Halperin J, Harbaugh R, Johnston SC, Katzan I, Kelly-Hayes M, Kenton EJ, Marks M, Schwamm LH, Tomsick T, American Heart Association, American Stroke Association Council on Stroke, Council on Cardiovascular Radiology and Intervention, American Academy of Neurology: Guidelines for prevention of stroke in patients with ischemic stroke or transient ischemic attack: a statement for healthcare professionals from the American Heart Association/American Stroke Association Council on Stroke: co-sponsored by the Council on Cardiovascular Radiology and Intervention: the American Academy of Neurology affirms the value of this guideline. Stroke 2006;37:577–617.
19 Adams RJ, Albers GW, Alberts, MJ, Benavente O, Furie K, Goldstein LB, Gorelick P, Halperin J, Harbaugh R, Johnston SC, Katzan I, Kelly-Hayes M, Kenton EJ, Marks M, Sacco RL, Schwamm LH: Update to the AHA/ASA Recommendations for the prevention of stroke in patients with stroke and transient ischemic attack. Stroke 2008;39:1647–1652.
20 Furie KL, Kasner SE, Adams RJ, Albers GW, Bush RL, Fagan SC, Halperin JL, Johnston SC, Katzan I, Kernan WN, Mitchell PH, Ovbiagele B, Palesch YY, Sacco RL, Schwamm LH, Wassertheil-Smoller S, Turan TN, Wentworth D, the American Heart Association Stroke Council, Council on Cardiovascular Nursing, Council on Clinical Cardiology, and Interdisciplinary Council on Quality of Care and Outcomes Research: Guidelines for the prevention of stroke in patients with stroke or transient ischemic attack: a guideline for healthcare professionals from the American Heart Association/American Stroke Association. Stroke 2011;42:227–276.
21 The European Stroke Organization (ESO) Executive Committee and the ESO Writing Committee: Guidelines for management of ischaemic stroke and transient ischaemic attack 2008. Cerebrovasc Dis 2008; 25:457–507.

22 Lansberg MG, O'Donnell MJ, Khatri P, Lang ES, Nguyen-Huynh MN, Schwartz NE, Sonnenberg FA, Schulman S, Vandvik PO, Spencer FA, Alonso-Coello P, Guyatt GH, Akl EA: Antithrombotic and thrombolytic therapy for ischemic stroke. Antithrombotic therapy and prevention of thrombosis, ed 9: American College of Chest Physicians Evidence-Based Clinical Practice Guidelines. Chest 2012;141:e601S–e636S.

23 Furie KL, Goldstein LB, Albers GW, Khatri P, Neyens R, Turakhia MP, Turan TN, Wood KA, the American Heart Association Stroke Council, Council on Quality of Care and Outcomes Research, Council on Cardiovascular Nursing, Council on Clinical Cardiology, and Council on Peripheral Vascular Disease: Oral antithrombotic agents for the prevention of stroke in nonvalvular atrial fibrillation: a science advisory for healthcare professionals from the American Heart Association/American Stroke Association. The American Academy of Neurology affirms the value of this statement as an educational tool for neurologists. Stroke, DOI: 10.1161/STR.0b013e318266722a.

24 Camm AJ, Lip GYH, De Caterina R, Savelieva I, Dan Atar D, Hohnloser SH, Hindricks G, Kirchhof P: An update of the 2010 ESC Guidelines for the management of atrial fibrillation. Developed with the special contribution of the European Heart Rhythm Association. http://www.escardio.org/guidelines.

25 Special report from the National Institute of Neurological Disorders and Stroke. Classification of cerebrovascular diseases III. Stroke 1990;21:637–676.

26 Uchiyama S: New definition and concept of TIA. Clin Neurol 2010;50:904–906.

27 Sorensen AG, Ay H: Transient ischemic attack: definition, diagnosis, and risk stratification. Neuroimaging Clin N Am 2011;21:303–313.

28 Johnston SC, Rothwell PM, Nguyen-Huynh MN, Giles MF, Elkins JS, Bernstein AL, Sidney S: Validation and refinement of scores to predict very early stroke risk after transient ischaemic attack. Lancet 2007;369:283–292.

29 Giles MF, Albers GW, Amarenco P, Arsava MM, Asimos A, Ay H, Calvet D, Coutts S, Cucchiara BL, Demchuk AM, Johnston SC, Kelly PJ, Kim AS, Labreuche J, Lavallee PC, Mas JL, Merwick A, Olivot JM, Purroy F, Rosamond WD, Sciolla R, Rothwell PM: Addition of brain infarction to the ABCD2 Score (ABCD^{2}I): a collaborative analysis of unpublished data on 4,574 patients. Stroke 2010;41:1907–1913.

30 Warrior L, Prabhakaran P: Transient ischemic attack evaluation models: hospitalization, same-day clinics, or rapid evaluation units. Am J Ther 2011;18:45–50.

Toshiyuki Uehara
National Cerebral and Cardiovascular Center
5-7-1 Fujishirodai
Suita, Osaka 565-8565 (Japan)
E-Mail tuehara@hsp.ncvc.go.jp

Uchiyama S, Amarenco P, Minematsu K, Wong KSL (eds): TIA as Acute Cerebrovascular Syndrome.
Front Neurol Neurosci. Basel, Karger, 2014, vol 33, pp 115–122 (DOI: 10.1159/000351913)

Radiological Examinations of Transient Ischemic Attack

Christie E. Tung · Jean Marc Olivot · Gregory W. Albers

Stanford University Medical Center, Palo Alto, Calif., USA

Abstract

Neuroimaging is critical in the evaluation of patients with TIA. CT and MRI are the two available options for imaging. Head CT is more widely available and commonly used. Diffusion MRI is the recommended modality to image an ischemic lesion. The presence of a diffusion lesion in a patient with transient neurological symptoms is an indicator of a high risk of recurrent stroke. Perfusion imaging with perfusion MRI or CT perfusion may improve the detection of ischemic lesions. Noninvasive vessel imaging may detect a symptomatic vessel lesion associated with an increased risk of stroke.

In 2009, the American Heart Association, the American Stroke Association, and the American Academy of Neurology endorsed a new definition of TIA. A transient episode of neurological dysfunction caused by focal brain, spinal cord or retinal ischemia without acute infarction. Stroke is now defined as a symptomatic infarction of the central nervous system tissue. This tissue-based definition has several implications. First, patients with transient neurological symptoms may have acute infarction of the brain. Second, diffusion-weighted imaging (DWI), the most sensitive imaging modality to confirm the diagnosis of infarction, becomes a critical tool in the evaluation of patients presenting with transient neurological symptoms of presumed ischemic mechanism [1].

The first obstacle a clinician has to overcome is how to confirm the ischemic mechanism of transient neurological symptoms when several non-ischemic pathologies can mimic TIA. Population studies indicate that about 5% of TIA patients suffer a stroke within 2 days of symptom onset. Urgent assessment and management of TIA can drastically reduce the risk of stroke. Therefore, patients with symptoms compatible with a TIA should undergo an urgent diagnostic evaluation.

Several studies have demonstrated substantial lack of agreement regarding TIA diagnosis among emergency department (ED) physicians, neurologists and even stroke specialists, whose judgment is often considered as the gold standard [2, 3]. Substantial disagreements regarding TIA diagnosis imply that patients with transient neurologic symptoms are at high risk to receive either inadequate or unnecessary treatments. Brain imaging can help the physician to clarify TIA diagnosis.

When the diagnosis of a TIA is made, the clinician should stratify the individual risk profile of the patient. The $ABCD^2$ score refers to clinical characteristics associated with an increased risk of stroke: age, blood pressure, type and duration of symptoms and the presence of diabetes [4]. The $ABCD^2$ score has performed well in epidemiological studies, but recent data strongly suggest that some patients with a low $ABCD^2$ score may have a high risk of stroke [5]. In 2010, our group participated in 2 pooled analyses which evaluated the benefits of including brain and vessel imaging findings in conjunction with the $ABCD^2$ score to improve risk assessment in TIA patients [5, 6]. Both studies demonstrated that the incorporation of imaging results improved the predictive power of the score.

Imaging an Ischemic Lesion

Computed Tomography

The most common imaging technique used for the evaluation of acute TIA is non-contrast head CT. CT imaging is widely available and can be rapidly performed in most EDs. It can be performed in patients with MR contraindications such as claustrophobia and metal implants. Several hours after the onset of ischemia, decreased density of the brain tissue on non-contrast head CT may reveal acute infarction.

Given the short duration of ischemia in TIA, the detection of an acute ischemic lesion on a non-contrast head CT is low, and in a retrospective study an ischemic lesion was found on non-contrast CT in less than 4% of TIA patients [7]. A recent meta-analysis of 1,368 TIA patients documented 327 (24%) with evidence of prior infarction (acute and chronic) on CT [6]. Infarction on CT increased the risk of stroke to 12.8% within 7 days compared to 9% in the CT-negative group, and improved the predictive power of the $ABCD^2$ score for early recurrent stroke [6, 8]. Although the accuracy of non-contrast head CT for the diagnosis of TIA is low, indirect markers of brain ischemia (i.e. the presence of chronic infarcts) may help the physician predict the risk of stroke after a TIA.

CT perfusion (CTP) imaging has developed concurrently with MR perfusion imaging and is now available for the evaluation of acute TIA patient. CTP can be performed in sequence with other techniques, such as CT angiography. Recent advances in CT technology (128 or 256 slice scanners) offer improved brain coverage. In one study, CTP was positive in 35% (12/34) of TIA patients [9]. In another small single-center study evaluating CTP in TIA patients, an acute ischemic lesion was found in 22 (34%) of 65 patients with motor and/or speech TIA symptoms [10]. This study also suggested that the presence of an ischemic lesion detected on CTP was associated with an increased risk of future stroke. This result remains to be confirmed in a large prospective study.

In conclusion, CT with or without CTP is a reasonable approach for the evaluation of TIA patients when MRI is contraindicated or not available. A systematic evaluation of a multimodal CT approach for the evaluation of patients with TIA is needed.

Magnetic Resonance

MRI has several advantages over CT. It can detect acute ischemic changes sooner than CT, and it has greater interobserver and intraobserver reliability than CT. Intracranial hemorrhage can be detected on MRI as easily as on CT [11]. Multimodal MRI is more specific and sensitive than head CT for the detection of acute ischemia [11]. DWI reveals an acute infarction in 30% of patients with a discharge diagnosis of TIA [6, 8, 11–14]. Symptom characteristics (motor deficit or speech disorder) and the presence of a symptomatic vessel lesion are associated with the presence of an acute ischemic lesion on DWI [15].

Several studies have shown that DWI positivity has prognostic implications. A recent meta-analysis showed that 7% of TIA patients with a positive DWI will suffer a stroke within a week compared to only 0.5% of the DWI-negative patients [6]. Interestingly, in DWI-negative patients the $ABCD^2$ score did not influence the risk of stroke, suggesting that a proportion of these patients may not have experienced a transient ischemic event [8]. By comparison, patients with a negative head CT still have an increased risk of stroke stratified by the $ABCD^2$ score. Because of the sensitivity of DWI in detecting brain infarction in TIA patients, DWI is recommended in the emergent evaluation of every TIA patient [15].

Two types of automatically processed MR perfusion sequences are now available: dynamic susceptibility contrast (DSC) perfusion-weighted imaging (PWI) and arterial spin labeling (ASL) perfusion imaging. DSC PWI is the most widely used perfusion modality. It requires a bolus contrast injection and is contraindicated in patients with renal insufficiency [16]. Fully automated software provides reliable and quantitative processing of DSC perfusion maps, making them available for review within 5 min of MRI completion [17]. Our group studied the presence of ischemic lesions on DSC PWI in a cohort of 69 unselected consecutive patients referred for suspicion of TIA [9]. PWI revealed an ischemic lesion in 33% of the patients. Half of the PWI-positive patients had a negative DWI. Most of the ischemic lesions on PWI were detected in the absence of vessel stenosis or occlusion on magnetic resonance angiography (MRA), which may reflect a distal occlusion not captured by MRA or no-reflow phenomenon. Another study prospectively evaluated TIA and minor stroke in patients with baseline perfusion deficits. MRI performed one week

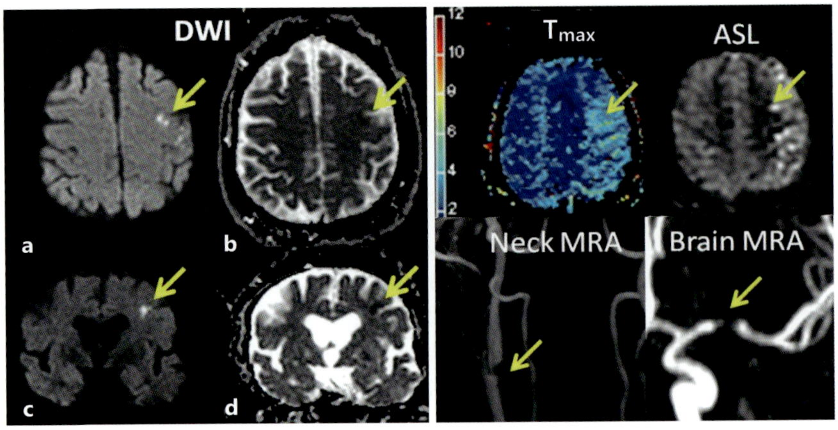

Fig. 1. Examples of MRI lesions. Diffusion: increased signal on B1000 axial A and coronal C with decreased signal on ADC (B and D). PWI T_{max}: increased T_{max} delay in the left MCA territory. ASL: Hypersignal demonstrating slow flow in the left MCA territory. Cervical MRA with contrast: left panel 70% ICA stenosis. Brain MRA: right panel MCA stenosis.

later documented the development of new DWI lesions in the regions of initial perfusion deficit [18].

ASL perfusion imaging enables measurement of cerebral blood flow using a diffusible tracer: magnetically labeled water. Therefore, ASL can be performed in every patient eligible for a brain MRI. The strong dependence of the ASL signal on the arterial arrival time may explain its sensitivity to detect transient and minor hypoperfusion lesions that accompany TIAs [19]. We studied the yield of ASL in a cohort of 76 patients referred for suspicion of TIA [9]. The inter-rater agreement was similar to that observed with DSC PWI. ASL was positive in 35% of those who had a final diagnosis of TIA. Half of the patients with an ischemic lesion detected by ASL were DWI negative. Fifty-five patients underwent both DSC and ASL perfusion imaging. Using both techniques, positive lesions were found in 53% of those who had a final diagnosis of TIA. These results suggest that the techniques are complementary for the detection of an ischemic lesion in TIA patients and that ASL can be performed in place of bolus perfusion when it is not available or contraindicated (see fig. 1). MR perfusion imaging may be positive in other situations than TIAs. Chronic infarctions are frequently hypoperfused and may cause seizures that can be confused for TIAs. Micro- and macrobleeds may also contaminate GRE-based perfusion maps and cause seizures that can be misinterpreted as TIAs [20]. MR perfusion abnormalities have also been associated with severe migraine with aura [21].

Despite the large number of clinical studies and guidelines suggesting the benefits of MRI, the proportion of TIA patients evaluated by MRI in North America during the last decade remained very low (<10%) [22, 23]. Even among some of most of the advanced TIA centers, only 40% of TIA patients underwent an MRI within 24 h after symptom onset [5].

Vessel Imaging

In addition to brain imaging, the American Heart Association statement on the definition and evaluation of TIA calls for noninvasive imaging of the craniocervical vessels [1]. Computed tomography angiography (CTA), MRA, or sonographic evaluation (carotid ultrasound/transcranial Doppler) are recommended, although there is no preferred method of vessel imaging. Sonography is discussed in detail in another chapter of this publication. The importance of vessel imaging in the evaluation and management of TIA was recently confirmed in the CATCH study [24]. Positive CTA (occlusion or stenosis ≥50% in the intracranial or extracranial vessels on the clinically relevant side) was an independent predictor of recurrent stroke. The hazard ratio of 4 for positive CT/CTA in CATCH was consistent with that reported in a prior study for moderate-to-severe large artery disease defined by ultrasound [25]. Vessel occlusion on MRA is also associated with a 4-fold increased risk of stroke [26]. Regarding the intracranial vessels, the sensitivity and specificity of CTA for detecting ≥50% stenosis is 95% [25]. The sensitivity and specificity of 3-D time-of-flight MRA is approximately 90% [27]. In the extracranial vessels, the sensitivity and specificity of both CTA and contrast MRA are about 90% for severe disease (≥70%), making them roughly equivalent for detecting severe disease. However, for moderate (50–69%) stenosis, the sensitivity and specificity of MRA drops to 66 and 94% according to recent systematic review [28]. CTA is more widely available and can be quickly performed. Because it requires contrast dye, use of CTA is limited in patients with dye allergies and renal failure, and in these cases MRA may be sufficient. There have been no direct studies comparing combined CT/CTA and DWI/MRA.

Imaging Strategies

In accordance with the American Heart Association guidelines and the above presented data, urgent neuroimaging within 24 h of the onset of symptoms is recommended for the evaluation of patients with presumed TIA [1]. MRI is the recommended imaging technique for the evaluation of TIA patients. However, in cases where MRI is not available or it is contraindicated, CT should be performed. Noninvasive imaging of the intracranial and extracranial vessels (CTA, MRA) may be performed during CT and MRI brain imaging or by ultrasound.

At Stanford, the evaluation of TIA patients referred to our ED includes a systematic MRI protocol performed within 12 h after patient arrival. The sequences recommended are DWI, MRA of the head and neck, DSC PWI, and ASL. If patients cannot receive gadolinium contrast, we obtain MRI with ASL perfusion, MRA of the head, and time-of-flight MRA of the neck (see fig. 2). In patients with MRI contraindications, non-contrast CT with CTA and CTP is obtained. Finally, cervical and transcra-

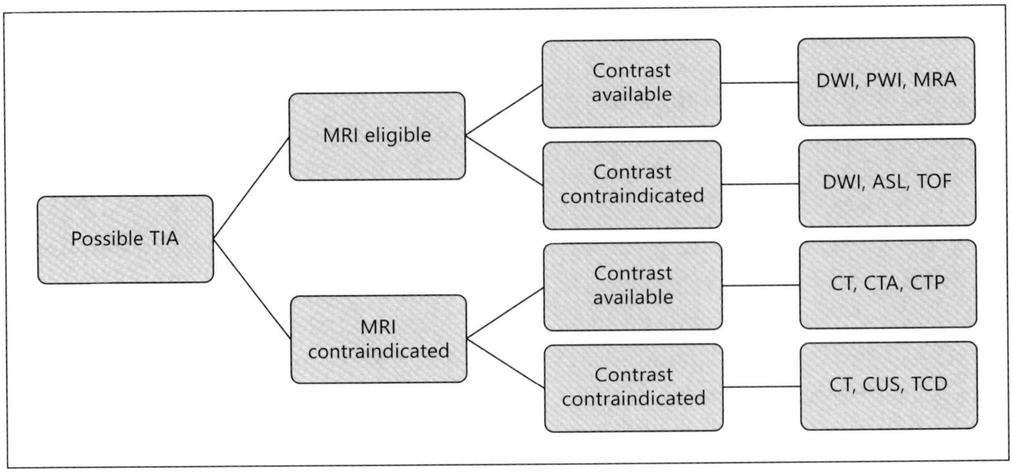

Fig. 2. Stanford TIA imaging strategy. MRI is contraindicated when MR is incompatible with metal implant or device. Contrast is contraindicated when renal impairment or contrast allergy is present. TOF = Time of flight; CUS = carotid ultrasound; TCD = transcranial Doppler.

nial Doppler are recommended when iodinated contrast is contraindicated. In a recent cohort of 129 patients evaluated in the ED for acute TIA, 112 (92%) underwent an MRI after a median delay of 8.2 h from arrival and 15.7 h from symptom onset [unpubl. data; 29].

Conclusion

The use of multimodal MRI has dramatically changed the evaluation of TIA patients. The detection of an acute ischemic lesion on diffusion and/or perfusion imaging in 50% of TIA patients helps the physician to confirm an ischemic mechanism for transient neurological symptoms. In addition, the presence of an infarction on DWI redefines TIA as a brain infarction with transient neurological symptoms and is associated in retrospective studies with a high risk of recurrent stroke. In addition, noninvasive vessel imaging may reveal the presence of a symptomatic intracranial or cervical vessel lesion that is associated with an increased risk of recurrent stroke. When MRI is contraindicated, non-contrast CT coupled with CTA and CTP, or ultrasound imaging, are acceptable alternatives for the evaluation of TIA patients.

References

1 Easton JD, Saver JL, Albers GW, Alberts MJ, Chaturvedi S, Feldmann E, Hatsukami TS, Higashida RT, Johnston SC, Kidwell CS, Lutsep HL, Miller E, Sacco RL: Definition and evaluation of transient ischemic attack: a scientific statement for healthcare professionals from the American Heart Association/American Stroke Association Stroke Council; Council on Cardiovascular Surgery and Anesthesia; Council on Cardiovascular Radiology and Intervention; Council on Cardiovascular Nursing; and the Interdisciplinary Council on Peripheral Vascular Disease. The American Academy of Neurology affirms the value of this statement as an educational tool for neurologists. Stroke 2009;40:2276–2293.

2 Prabhakaran S, Silver AJ, Warrior L, McClenathan B, Lee VH: Misdiagnosis of transient ischemic attacks in the emergency room. Cerebrovasc Dis 2008;26: 630–635.

3 Castle J, Mlynash M, Lee K, Caulfield AF, Wolford C, Kemp S, Hamilton S, Albers GW, Olivot JM: Agreement regarding diagnosis of transient ischemic attack fairly low among stroke-trained neurologists. Stroke 2010;41:1367–1370.

4 Johnston SC, Rothwell PM, Nguyen-Huynh MN, Giles MF, Elkins JS, Bernstein AL, Sidney S: Validation and refinement of scores to predict very early stroke risk after transient ischaemic attack. Lancet 2007;369:283–292.

5 Merwick A, Albers GW, Amarenco P, Arsava EM, Ay H, Calvet D, Coutts SB, Cucchiara BL, Demchuk AM, Furie KL, Giles MF, Labreuche J, Lavallee PC, Mas JL, Olivot JM, Purroy F, Rothwell PM, Saver JL, Sheehan OC, Stack JP, Walsh C, Kelly PJ: Addition of brain and carotid imaging to the ABCD(2) score to identify patients at early risk of stroke after transient ischaemic attack: a multicentre observational study. Lancet Neurol 2010;9:1060–1069.

6 Giles MF, Albers GW, Amarenco P, Arsava MM, Asimos A, Ay H, Calvet D, Coutts S, Cucchiara BL, Demchuk AM, Johnston SC, Kelly PJ, Kim AS, Labreuche J, Lavallee PC, Mas JL, Merwick A, Olivot JM, Purroy F, Rosamond WD, Sciolla R, Rothwell PM: Addition of brain infarction to the ABCD2 Score (ABCD2I): a collaborative analysis of unpublished data on 4574 patients. Stroke 2010;41:1907–1913.

7 Douglas VC, Johnston CM, Elkins J, Sidney S, Gress DR, Johnston SC: Head computed tomography findings predict short-term stroke risk after transient ischemic attack. Stroke 2003;34:2894–2898.

8 Giles MF, Albers GW, Amarenco P, Arsava MM, Asimos A, Ay H, Calvet D, Coutts SB, Cucchiara BL, Demchuk AM, Johnston SC, Kelly PJ, Kim AS, Labreuche J, Lavallee PC, Mas JL, Merwick A, Olivot JM, Purroy F, Rosamond WD, Sciolla R, Rothwell PM: Early stroke risk and ABCD2 score performance in tissue- vs time-defined TIA: a multicenter study. Neurology 2011;77:1222–1228.

9 Kleinman JT, Zaharchuk G, Mlynash M, Ogdie AA, Straka M, Lansberg MG, Schwartz NE, Kemp S, Bammer R, Albers GW, Olivot JM: Automated perfusion imaging for the evaluation of transient ischemic attack. Stroke 2012;43:1556–1560.

10 Prabhakaran S, Patel SK, Samuels J, McClenathan B, Mohammad Y, Lee VH: Perfusion computed tomography in transient ischemic attack. Arch Neurol 2011;68:85–89.

11 Chalela JA, Kidwell CS, Nentwich LM, Luby M, Butman JA, Demchuk AM, Hill MD, Patronas N, Latour L, Warach S: Magnetic resonance imaging and computed tomography in emergency assessment of patients with suspected acute stroke: a prospective comparison. Lancet 2007;369:293–298.

12 Ay H, Arsava EM, Johnston SC, Vangel M, Schwamm LH, Furie KL, Koroshetz WJ, Sorenson AG: Clinicaland imaging-based prediction of stroke risk after transient ischemic attack: the CIP model. Stroke 2009;40:181–186.

13 Redgrave JN, Coutts SB, Schulz UG, Briley D, Rothwell PM: Systematic review of associations between the presence of acute ischemic lesions on diffusion-weighted imaging and clinical predictors of early stroke risk after transient ischemic attack. Stroke 2007;38:1482–1488.

14 Redgrave JN, Schulz UG, Briley D, Meagher T, Rothwell PM: Presence of acute ischaemic lesions on diffusion-weighted imaging is associated with clinical predictors of early risk of stroke after transient ischaemic attack. Cerebrovasc Dis 2007;24:86–90.

15 Purroy F, Montaner J, Rovira A, Delgado P, Quintana M, Alvarez-Sabín J: Higher risk of further vascular events among transient ischemic attack patients with diffusion-weighted imaging acute ischemic lesions. Stroke 2004;35:2313–2319.

16 Calamante F, Gadian DG, Connelly A: Quantification of perfusion using bolus tracking magnetic resonance imaging in stroke: assumptions, limitations, and potential implications for clinical use. Stroke 2002;33:1146–1151.

17 Straka M, Albers GW, Bammer R: Real-time diffusion-perfusion mismatch analysis in acute stroke. J Magn Reson Imaging 2010;32:1024–1037.

18 Asdaghi N, Bilal H, Saini M, Emery D, Jeerakathil T, Butcher K: Acute perfusion and diffusion abnormalities predict early new MRI lesions one week after minor stroke and TIA. Stroke 2011;42:2191–2195.
19 Zaharchuk G: Arterial spin label imaging of acute ischemic stroke and transient ischemic attack. Neuroimaging Clin N Am 2011;21:285–301.
20 Viswanathan A, Chabriat H: Cerebral microhemorrhage. Stroke 2006;37:550–555.
21 Kapinos G, Fischbein NJ, Zaharchuk G, Venkatasubramanian C: Migraine-like headache with visual deficit and perfusion abnormality on MRI. Neurology 2010;74:1743–1745.
22 Gladstone DJ, Kapral MK, Fang J, Laupacis A, Tu JV: Management and outcomes of transient ischemic attacks in Ontario. CMAJ 2004;170:1099–1104.
23 Edlow JA, Kim S, Pelletier AJ, Camargo CA Jr: National study on emergency department visits for transient ischemic attack, 1992–2001. Acad Emerg Med 2006;13:666–672.
24 Coutts SB, Modi J, Patel SK, Demchuk AM, Goyal M, Hill MD, Calgary Stroke Program: CT/CT angiography and MRI findings predict recurrent stroke after transient ischemic attack and minor stroke: results of the prospective CATCH study. Stroke 2012;43: 1013–1017.
25 Nguyen-Huynh MN, Wintermark M, English J, Lam J, Vittinghoff E, Smith WS, Johnston SC: How accurate is CT angiography in evaluating intracranial atherosclerotic disease? Stroke 2008;39:1184–1188.
26 Coutts SB, Simon JE, Eliasziw M, Sohn CH, Hill MD, Barber PA, Palumbo V, Kennedy J, Roy J, Gagnon A, Scott JN, Buchan AM, Demchuk AM: Triaging transient ischemic attack and minor stroke patients using acute magnetic resonance imaging. Ann Neurol 2005;57:848–854.
27 Hirai T, Korogi Y, Ono K, Nagano M, Maruoka K, Uemura S, Takahashi M: Prospective evaluation of suspected stenoocclusive disease of the intracranial artery: combined MR angiography and CT angiography compared with digital subtraction angiography. Am J Neuroradiol 2002;23:93–101.
28 Debrey SM, Yu H, Lynch JK, Lovblad KO, Wright VL, Janket SJ, Baird AE: Diagnostic accuracy of magnetic resonance angiography for internal carotid artery disease: a systematic review and meta-analysis. Stroke 2008;39:2237–2248.
29 Vora N, Tung CE, Mlynash M, Waimei T, Garcia M, Kemp S, Albers GW, Olivot JM: Magnetic resonance imaging based transient ischemic attack triage in the emergency department is feasible and safe; in Int Stroke Conf, New Orleans, February 2012.

Christie E. Tung, MD
Stanford University Medical Center
780 Welch Rd, Suite 205
Palo Alto, CA 94304 (USA)
E-Mail cetung@stanford.edu

Uchiyama S, Amarenco P, Minematsu K, Wong KSL (eds): TIA as Acute Cerebrovascular Syndrome.
Front Neurol Neurosci. Basel, Karger, 2014, vol 33, pp 123–134 (DOI: 10.1159/000353193)

Neurosonological Examinations of Transient Ischemic Attack

Vijay K. Sharma[a] • K.S. Lawrence Wong[b]

[a]Division of Neurology, National University Hospital, Singapore, Singapore; [b]Division of Neurology, Prince of Wales Hospital, Chinese University of Hong Kong, Hong Kong, SAR, China

Abstract

Cerebrovascular ultrasonography is the only modality that provides real-time information about blood flow in various cervicocerebral arteries. Continuous information can be obtained over extended periods with high resolution and excellent spatial display. Hemodynamic changes in the cerebral circulation due to various physiological or pathological states can be monitored reliably. The information obtained from cerebrovascular ultrasonography carries diagnostic, therapeutic as well as prognostic potential in various conditions. Cervical duplex sonography evaluates blood flow as well as arterial wall characteristics in the major arteries that supply the cerebral vascular bed. Validated criteria for the diagnosis of steno-occlusive disease of carotid or vertebral arteries have high accuracy parameters. Transcranial Doppler (TCD) ultrasonography provides a reliable evaluation of intracranial blood flow patterns in real-time and adds physiological information to the anatomical details obtained from other neuroimaging modalities. Cerebrovascular ultrasonography is relatively cheap, can be performed at bedside, and allows monitoring in acute emergency settings. Extended applications of TCD provide important information about the pathophysiology of cerebrovascular ischemia and risk stratification. Therefore, cerebrovascular ultrasonography has become an integral component of the armamentarium of stroke neurologists for understanding stroke etiopathogenesis, planning and monitoring definitive treatment and determining the prognosis. It has been suggested as an essential component of a comprehensive stroke center. We have reviewed various established applications of ultrasonography in patients with cerebrovascular ischemia.

Transient ischemic attack (TIA) is often considered as a medical emergency that carries a substantial short-term risk of acute ischemic stroke [1, 2]. Recent advances in imaging technology have significantly improved our understanding of the etiopathophysiology of TIA. The current guidelines advocate the urgent diagnostic evaluation of all TIA patients and immediate hospitalization of high-risk cases [3].

Owing to the limited availability, risk of radiation exposure with various imaging modalities, cost and risk of nephrotoxicity with contrast agents, noninvasive imaging methods with acceptable accuracy parameters for determining the degree of arterial stenosis in cervicocerebral arteries are the preferred methods for initial screening of patients with acute cerebrovascular ischemia. Furthermore, cerebrovascular ultrasound helps in the evaluation of suspicious findings on physical examination (for example, bruits). Although vascular imaging is urgently indicated in TIA, it is not performed in time in a significant proportion of patients. Availability of diagnostic imaging methods and their cost remain the commonest limiting factors, especially in the developing world. These limitations can be overcome, at least to some extent, by using cerebrovascular ultrasonography as the primary screening modality. In addition to confirming the focal cerebral ischemia as the cause of TIA due to various steno-occlusive diseases of the cervicocerebral arterial tree, cerebrovascular ultrasonography might help in identifying suitable patients for various therapeutic interventions. While cervical duplex ultrasonography (CDU) can evaluate major arteries in the neck, transcranial Doppler (TCD) would help in understanding various hemodynamic adjustments in patients with steno-occlusive disease of cervicocerebral arteries. In this article, we would discuss the basic principles of CDU and TCD along with their advanced application in specific steno-occlusive disease states.

Cervical Duplex Ultrasonography

CDU is widely used in patients with cerebrovascular ischemia to screen the extracranial carotid and vertebral occlusive diseases [3]. CDU is relatively cheap and a bedside tool that provides important information regarding the status of vascular lumen and atherosclerotic burden in major cervical arteries. Currently available carotid imaging modalities (digital subtraction angiography, magnetic resonance angiography and computerized tomographic angiography) provide information about the arterial lumen only. CDU possesses a unique ability to evaluate the arterial wall as well as the lumen. Hence, it can be used to evaluate atherosclerotic disease burden by carotid wall imaging for intima-media thickness (IMT) and atheromatous plaques as well as for luminal imaging to estimate the degree of stenosis.

IMT is measured as the distance between lumen/intima interface to the media/adventitia interface and an increased IMT is considered the earliest sign of carotid atherosclerosis. It can be measured either manually or by inbuilt software in some ultrasound scanners. An atheromatous plaque is described as a focal increase in the IMT (more than 1.2 mm). Carotid plaques are described by their composition (echogenicity) and surface. The pivotal Tromso study showed that echolucent plaques are associated with increased risk of cerebrovascular events, independent of the degree of stenosis and other cardiovascular risk factors [4]. Hypo- or anechogenic plaques and plaques with complex pattern of echogenicity carry higher risk of cerebrovascular

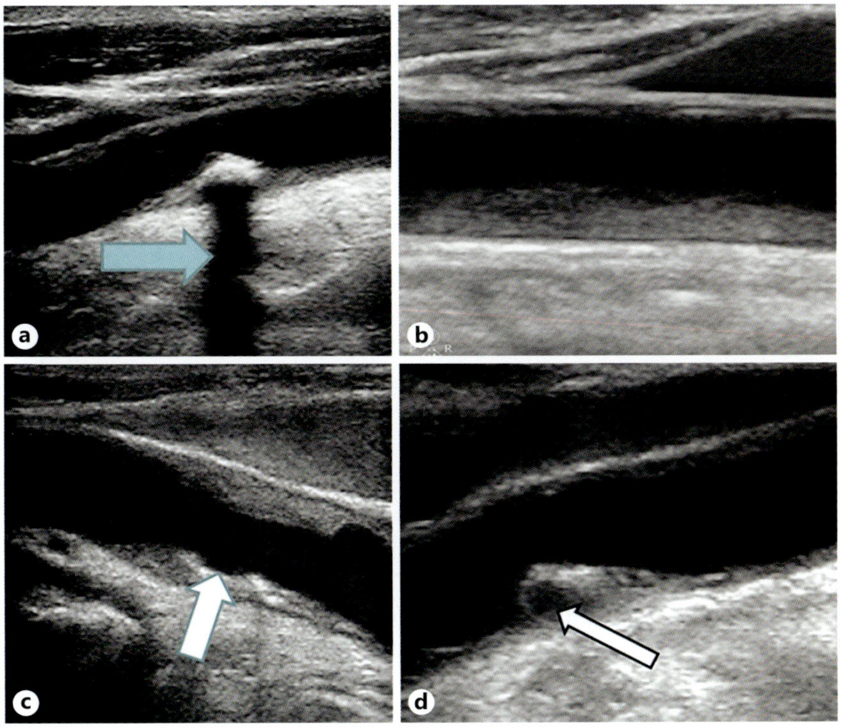

Fig. 1. Brightness mode (B-mode) images of carotid artery and various types of plaques. **a** A calcified plaque produces a dense shadow (arrow) behind due to strong reflection. Tissues behind the calcified plaques cannot be evaluated due to this intense shadow. **b** A large smooth homogeneous plaque is noted. **c** Ulceration of a plaque (arrow) seen as a breach on the surface of the plaque increases the risk of local thrombus formation and distal embolization. **d** Sometimes the atherosclerotic plaque grows bigger, and an area can break down due to necrosis and intraplaque hemorrhage, considered to be associated with significantly higher risk of distal embolization and ischemic stroke.

events than echogenic and heterogeneous plaques [5]. Various types of plaques seen on CDU are shown in figure 1. The plaque is usually covered by a thin hyperintense rim of fibrous tissue, while 'ulceration' corresponds to an irregularity or break in its surface. A significant ulcerations recess must be at least 2 mm deep and 2 mm long. Carotid plaque surface irregularity/ulceration exposes the thrombogenic layers, leading to thrombus formation and embolization. The guidelines for selecting the high-risk patients remain vaguely defined. Cerebral embolization from atherosclerotic plaques is determined by its 'embolic potential'. Therefore, detection of microembolic signals (MES) on TCD may serve as a surrogate marker for stroke risk and help in identifying high-risk plaques, their embolic potential, effect of medical therapy as well as deciding the timing of various revascularization procedures.

Degree of carotid stenosis is the most important predictor of cerebrovascular events. CDU is often the primary diagnostic modality for carotid stenosis. CDU criteria for quantifying carotid stenosis have been validated against contrast arteriography, and for a carotid stenosis of 50–99%, it has sensitivity and specificity between 90 and 95% [6]. CDU can be used to monitor the progression of carotid stenosis in asymptomatic patients. Furthermore, it can also be used to monitor the results of carotid revascularization procedures.

Although steno-occlusive disease of carotid artery contributes most to TIA, vertebral or subclavian arteries may also be involved in some cases. CDU permits reliable evaluation of these cervical arteries too.

Transcranial Doppler

TCD can be aptly called as the stethoscope for the brain. Since its introduction in 1982, TCD has evolved as a diagnostic, monitoring and therapeutic tool in patients with cerebrovascular ischemia. Currently, TCD is the only diagnostic tool that can provide real-time information about cerebral hemodynamics and can detect embolization to cerebral vessels. Similar to CDU, TCD is noninvasive and a bedside tool and helps in obtaining information regarding the collateral flow across various branches of the circle of Willis. Compared with computed tomography angiography, TCD has 79% sensitivity and 94% specificity in detecting intracranial stenosis [7]. Advanced applications of TCD like emboli monitoring, vasomotor reactivity and detection of right-to-left shunts (RLS) help in understating the etiopathogenesis of cerebrovascular ischemia, risk stratification and prognostication (fig. 2). In the setting of acute cerebrovascular ischemia, combined TCD and CDU can evaluate the cerebral hemodynamic consequences of extracranial carotid stenosis and help in identifying lesions amenable for interventional therapy [8].

Transcranial Color-Coded Duplex

Transcranial color-coded duplex (TCCD) provides two-dimensional gray-scale real-time and color Doppler imaging of the circle of Willis. It enables the operator to obtain angle-corrected flow velocities from various intracranial arterial segments.

TCCD might be considered more accurate in the assessment of flow velocities than conventional TCD. However, no direct comparison of both methods in pathologic conditions exists to date. The flow velocities in the intracranial arteries in healthy individuals are approximately 10–30% higher when measured using TCCD as compared to conventional TCD. The difference is believed to widen in patients with intracranial stenosis. The comparison of the diagnostic efficiency of both methods at the same velocity thresholds cannot be valid, and it is difficult to use the flow velocities defined by conventional TCD studies for analyzing intracranial stenosis by TCCD. TCCD has been reported to have high sensitivity and specificity in the detection of a

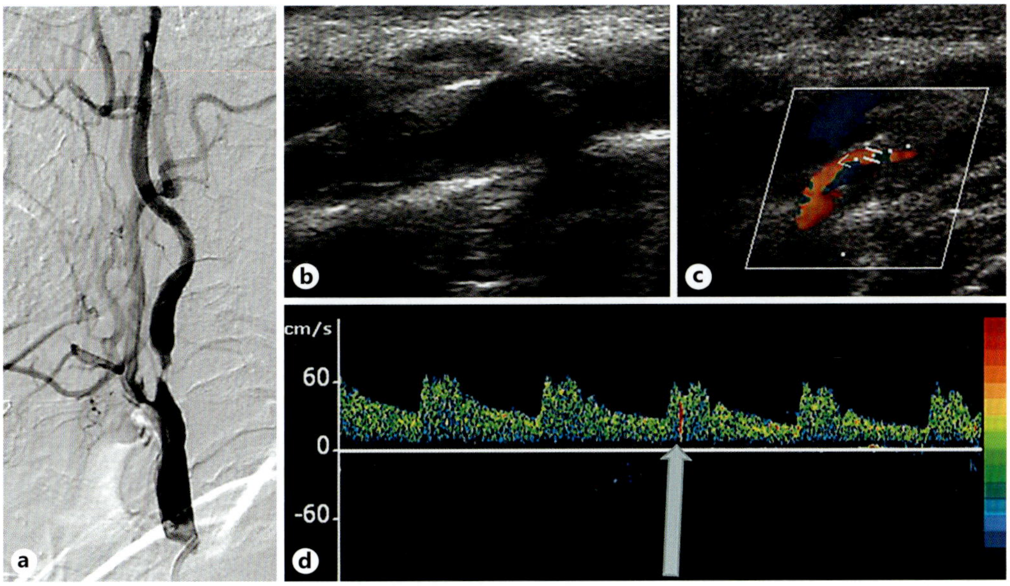

Fig. 2. Imaging and neurosonology findings in a patient with recurrent TIAs. This 67-year-old male presented with recurrent episodes of left-sided weakness for about one week. Magnetic resonance imaging of the brain was unremarkable. However, the magnetic resonance angiography demonstrated a severe focal stenosis of the proximal ICA in the neck, confirmed on digital subtraction angiography (**a**) and cervical duplex sonography (**b** and **c**). He continued to have recurrent episodes despite initiating aspirin. **d** TCD monitoring of the left MCA demonstrated spontaneous MES that disappeared upon starting dual antiplatelet therapy. The patient underwent a successful carotid endarterectomy after one week.

moderate intracranial stenosis. For instance, the WASID study used a mean flow velocity (MFV) threshold of 100 cm/s for middle cerebral artery (MCA) for TCD, considerably different when TCCD was used [9]. However, TCCD remains operator dependent, and the quality may be adversely affected in patients with insufficient temporal acoustic windows. Three-dimensional reconstruction during TCCD imaging and the use of sonographic contrast agents could help in improving the quality as well as reliability of the results.

Extracranial Carotid Stenosis

The internal carotid artery (ICA) stenosis is responsible for up to 20% of all cerebrovascular ischemic events, and the risk is proportional to the severity of stenosis. Severity of stenosis in the ICA unequivocally predicts the risk of stroke. Symptomatic hemodynamically significant stenosis in the ICA can cause cerebral ischemia due to thromboembolism or hemodynamic insufficiency.

Table 1. Diagnostic criteria for carotid stenosis

Degree of stenosis	ICA PSV, cm/s	ICA/CCA PSV ratio	ICA EDV, cm/s	Plaque
Normal	<125	<2.0	<40	none
<50%	<125	<2.0	<40	<50% diameter reduction
50–69%	125–230	2.0–4.0	40–100	>50% diameter reduction
70% to near occlusion	>230	>4.0	>100	>50% diameter reduction
Near occlusion	may be low or undetectable	variable	variable	a significantly reduced detectable lumen
Occlusion	undetectable	not applicable	not applicable	no detectable lumen

CCA = Common carotid artery; EDV = end-diastolic velocity.

Currently, detection of specific threshold levels of the ICA stenosis appears to be most clinically important, and the grading of carotid stenosis on CDU is based on the consensus criteria (table 1) [10]. Furthermore, various morphological characteristics of the carotid plaques have been described as determinants of their 'embolic potential'. In addition to the size of the plaque, these include plaque composition, intraplaque hemorrhage and ulceration on the surface [11].

Large randomized clinical trials have established the efficacy of endarterectomy (CEA) for the secondary prevention of stroke in patients with symptomatic ICA stenosis [12, 13]. These studies showed a 60–80% relative risk reduction, compared with best medical therapy in patients with symptomatic ICA stenosis ≥70%, provided the perioperative complication rates remained <7%, and surgery was performed within 2 weeks of symptoms. Although carotid angioplasty with stent placement (CAS) remains an alternative option to CEA, many clinical trials with CAS could not prove convincingly the non-inferiority, equivalence or superiority of CAS over CEA.

Carotid interventions require careful selection of suitable patients. TCD can play an important role in clinical decision-making by evaluating the hemodynamic effects of the carotid stenosis, detecting MES originating from the carotid plaque [14], identifying additional tandem lesions in the intracranial circulation and evaluation of vasomotor reactivity to identify symptomatic and asymptomatic patients at potentially high risk of stroke [15]. TCD is used at some centers for continuous monitoring of ipsilateral MCA flow as well as MES during carotid revascularization procedures. TCD can help in reducing the perioperative complications due to excessive embolization from the carotid plaque or cerebral hypoperfusion during cross-clamping as well as identifying patients with cerebral hyperperfusion syndrome after clam release [16]. Surveillance of the carotid artery after revascularization is essential since early as well as late recurrence of stenosis following successful operation is common.

TCD can help in medical management of patients with carotid stenosis. The Clopidogrel and Aspirin for Reduction of Emboli in Symptomatic Carotid Stenosis (CARESS) trial revealed that the combination of clopidogrel and aspirin was associated with a marked reduction in MES, compared with aspirin alone [17]. It has been found that in asymptomatic carotid stenosis, TCD-negative cases for microemboli do not benefit from carotid revascularization unless the procedural risk is <1%. It has been suggested that asymptomatic carotid stenosis should be managed medically, with delay of surgical intervention until the occurrence of symptoms or emboli [18].

Stenosis of Cervical Vertebral Arteries and Subclavian Steal Syndrome

Vertebro-basilar ischemia (VBI) accounts for about 20% of cerebral ischemic events and a delayed or incorrect diagnosis may result in serious morbidity or mortality [19]. Therefore, an urgent noninvasive neurovascular assessment of posterior circulation is critical for confirmation of vertebrobasilar steno-occlusive disease and identifying patients with poor prognosis and those who could benefit from possible interventions. Compared with contrast angiography, TCD has acceptable accuracy parameters (sensitivity 73%, specificity 96%, positive predictive value 68%, negative predictive value 95%, overall accuracy 93%) [20]. The circle of Willis may provide sufficient collateral pathways to perfuse the affected vascular territories in some patients with severe occlusive disease of the major cervicocerebral arteries. Accordingly, a reversed flow in the basilar artery, due to retrograde perfusion from the posterior communicating arteries, in patients with acute VBI is often associated with better clinical outcomes [20].

A blood pressure difference of >20 mm Hg between the two arms is often suggestive of subclavian artery stenosis. Such patients should undergo further diagnostic evaluation if VBI due to posterior circulation hypoperfusion is suspected. Subclavian steal syndrome (SSS) is usually an incidental finding and rarely causes VBI. It has been suggested that patients with SSS who develop VBI usually have additional steno-occlusive disease of intracranial or extracranial large arteries. Symptoms of cerebral ischemia due to SSS may be precipitated or aggravated in some patients by arm exercise. Reduced flow resistance due to exercise-induced vasodilation (hyperemia-ischemia cuff test) in the upper extremity might result in reduction of cerebral blood flow to critical levels in some patients, rendering them at higher risk of VBI.

TIAs due to regional cerebral hypoperfusion are uncommon and scarcely reported in the literature. The orthostatic TIAs typically occur with hemodynamically significant stenosis of a large artery, resulting in distal low perfusion states. TCD allows quantitative estimations of the changes in arterial flow velocity during orthostatic or position-induced ischemia [21].

Transcranial Doppler in Intracranial Stenosis

Intracranial arterial steno-occlusive lesions cause characteristic Doppler signals such as focal increases in flow velocities, turbulence, post-stenotic drop in velocity, blunted flow signals in distal segments and various collateral flow patterns. Intracranial stenosis may be seen in more than 50% of Asian patients with TIA [22]. The accuracy parameters of TCD are generally higher in anterior circulation than the vertebrobasilar circulation, owing to the more reliable anatomy of the former and technical problems in studying the latter [9]. However, the advent of PMD TCD has been reported with improved accuracy parameters, especially when the tests are performed early after the symptom onset and by experienced sonographers [21]. Diagnostic criteria for moderate stenosis in the intracranial arteries use highest cutoff velocities, either peak systolic flow velocity (PSV) or MFV or a combination of these two. Various cutoff values have been suggested. The flow velocities in MCAs are highest among all the intracranial arterial segments, and PSV above 140 cm/s or MFV more than 80 cm/s are considered to represent the presence of a moderate (more than 50%) focal stenosis. However, it is suggested that each laboratory should validate their findings against contrast angiography to determine the best cutoff values at their centers. There is an association between the degree of stenosis and recurrent stroke, with higher degrees of stenosis and the number of vessels affected having a worse prognosis [9, 22]. Wong et al. [23] reported that after adjustment for vascular risk factors and stroke severity, the adjusted odds ratio for various vascular events or death was 1.25 per occlusive artery (95% CI: 1.12–1.39). Furthermore, in a study of 705 patients, Wong and Li [24] observed higher incidence of stroke recurrence during the first year of diagnosis in patients with intracranial atherosclerosis (17.1 vs. 10.9% for patients without vascular lesion).

TCD can detect MES in TIA patients with stenosis of extracranial or intracranial stenosis and help in optimizing the antithrombotic therapy [17, 25]. The prospective CARESS study of 107 patients with symptomatic carotid disease and MES found fewer MES per hour and fewer strokes in patients treated with clopidogrel and aspirin than in patients treated with aspirin alone during the first week after symptom onset [17]. Similar reduction in the number of MES was noted with dual antiplatelet therapy in a randomized clinical trial in a patient population with intracranial large artery atherosclerosis [25].

Right-to-Left Shunt Detection

Patent foramen ovale (PFO) is common in general population with a prevalence of 10–35% in various echocardiography and autopsy studies. The prevalence could be much higher in certain selected populations, e.g. in patients with cryptogenic stroke or TIA and in younger patients without an apparent etiology. PFO with RLS is considered a potential risk factor for stroke in patients with stroke of unknown etiology. Although contrast-enhanced transesophageal echocardiography is considered as the gold standard for diagnosing PFO, TCD with agitated saline-air contrast mixture is a reliable method for detecting the presence of an RLS. The sensitivity and specificity of contrast TCD have been reported to be 68–100 and 67–100%, respectively [26]. Advantages of TCD include calibrated Valsalva maneuver and the ability to change body positioning during the test [27]. However, evidence about the best therapeutic option for preventing stroke in patients with RLS remains controversial. The recurrence rate of RLS-associated stroke has not been clearly established, and the few studies on secondary prevention have been unable to demonstrate an effective therapeutic strategy, i.e. antiplatelets, anticoagulation or PFO closure.

Vasomotor Reactivity

Cerebral autoregulation helps in maintaining the blood supply by compensating for changes in cerebral perfusion pressure. It enables constant cerebral blood flow over a wide range of systemic blood pressure by varying the diameter of the arteriolar sphincters. Vasomotor reactivity is the ability of the cerebral circulation to respond to vasomotor stimuli. This can be evaluated reliably with TCD by monitoring the real-time changes in the flow velocities in response to such stimuli. CO_2 levels in blood are the strongest determinants of blood flow, with increased levels of CO_2 causing vasodilatation and increasing cerebral blood flow. The ability to monitor both MCAs simultaneously makes TCD more reliable since the magnitude of vasodilatory challenge as well as all other physiological factors may be estimated with confidence by comparing the response in the atherosclerotic artery with the healthy MCA on the contralateral side. Markus and Harrison [28] described a simple measurement of the MCA velocity in response to 30 s of breath holding and termed it as Breath-Holding Index (BHI), calculated as

$$\mathrm{BHI} = \frac{\mathrm{MFV}_{\mathrm{end}} - \mathrm{MFV}_{\mathrm{baseline}}}{\mathrm{MFV}_{\mathrm{baseline}}} \times \frac{100}{\text{seconds of breath holding}}$$

A decreased BHI suggests failure of collateral flow to adapt to the stenosis progression. Therefore, impaired BHI can help identify patients at higher risk of stroke due to hypoperfusion in patients with severe steno-occlusive disease of ICA or MCA. Hypercapnia can paradoxically decrease the residual flow velocity in the affected vessel at the expected time of normal brain vasodilation when blood pool is shifted to nonischemic areas (intracranial steal phenomenon); this is described as 'reversed Robin Hood' syndrome with the analogy to 'rob the poor to feed the rich' in patients with acute cerebrovascular ischemia [29]. This steal is detectable and measurable by TCD.

Chernyshev et al. [8] evaluated the combined fast-track TCD and carotid/vertebral duplex to identify lesions amenable to interventional treatment (LAIT). LAIT was defined as occlusion, near occlusion, ≥50% stenosis or thrombi in an artery supplying brain area affected by ischemia. The current definition of LAIT may include chronic lesions, and caution should be exercised if these lesions are directly responsible for current symptoms in the patient. The yield and accuracy of ultrasound identification of LAIT is high, both in patients eligible as well as ineligible for thrombolysis. The sensitivity, specificity, positive and negative predictive values for TCD were observed as 96, 75, 96 and 75%, respectively. The corresponding values for carotid/vertebral duplex were 94, 90, 94 and 90%, respectively. The information obtained from cerebrovascular ultrasonography is complimentary to various angiographic evaluations in acute ischemic stroke.

In acute cerebrovascular ischemia, rapid localization of arterial occlusion on TCD can verify the vascular origin of the neurological deficit and indirectly judge the collateral blood supply compensating for an occlusion. Continuous or intermittent monitoring of the occlusions in large intracranial arteries can help in therapeutic decision-making for the next most efficient management steps such as further diagnostic or interventional procedures. A persistent large vessel occlusion or stenosis in patients with acute and spontaneously resolving deficits heralds a greater possibility for the patient's deterioration within the next 24 h. These TCD findings are also helpful in identifying patients with persisting arterial obstructions that will render the patient more vulnerable to blood pressure changes, head positioning, and inadequate hydration [30].

Ultrasound may also detect more than one occlusion present in the same patient, i.e. tandem lesions in the ICA and MCA, or VA and BA. These tandem lesions are detected by combining the information obtained from the Doppler spectra and collateral flow signals. For example, if a distal M1 MCA occlusion is present, it should produce antegrade flow diversion to anterior cerebral or posterior cerebral artery. If an additional obstruction exists in the proximal ICA, TCD will show anterior cross-filling via the anterior communicating artery, stenotic terminal ICA velocities, and/or reversed ophthalmic artery.

In conclusion, cerebrovascular ultrasonography and its extended applications play an important role in the management of patients with acute cerebrovascular ischemic episodes.

References

1 Giles MF, Rothwell PM: Transient ischaemic attack: clinical relevance, risk prediction and urgency of secondary prevention. Curr Opin Neurol 2009;22:46–53.

2 Tsivgoulis G, Stamboulis E, Sharma VK, Heliopoulos I, Voumvourakis K, Teoh HL, Patousi A, Andrikopoulou A, Lim EL, Stilou L, Sim TB, Chan BP, Stefanis L, Vadikolias K, Piperidou C: Multicenter external validation of the ABCD2 score in triaging TIA patients. Neurology 2010;74:1351–1357.

3 Easton JD, Saver JL, Albers GW, Alberts MJ, Chaturvedi S, Feldmann E, Hatsukami TS, Higashida RT, Johnston SC, Kidwell CS, Lutsep HL, Miller E, Sacco RL, American Heart Association, American Stroke Association Stroke Council, Council on Cardiovascular Surgery and Anesthesia, Council on Cardiovascular Radiology and Intervention, Council on Cardiovascular Nursing, Interdisciplinary Council on Peripheral Vascular Disease: Definition and evaluation of transient ischemic attack: a scientific statement for healthcare professionals from the American Heart Association/American Stroke Association Stroke Council; Council on Cardiovascular Surgery and Anesthesia; Council on Cardiovascular Radiology and Intervention; Council on Cardiovascular Nursing; and the Interdisciplinary Council on Peripheral Vascular Disease. The American Academy of Neurology affirms the value of this statement as an educational tool for neurologists. Stroke 2009;40:2276–2293.

4 Joakimsen O, Bønaa KH, Stensland-Bugge E: Reproducibility of ultrasound assessment of carotid plaque occurrence, thickness, and morphology. The Tromsø Study. Stroke 1997;28:2201–2207.

5 Johnson JM, Kennely M, Decesale D, Morgan S, Sparrow S: Natural history of asymptomatic plaque. Arch Surg 1985;120:1010–1012.

6 Colhoun E, MacErlean D: Carotid artery imaging using duplex scanning and bidirectional arteriography: a comparison. Clin Radiol 1984;35:101–106.

7 Tsivgoulis G, Sharma VK, Lao AY, Malkoff MD, Alexandrov AV: Validation of transcranial Doppler with computed tomography angiography in acute cerebral ischemia. Stroke 2007;38:1245–1249.

8 Chernyshev OY, Garami Z, Calleja S, Song J, Campbell MS, Noser EA, Shaltoni H, Chen CI, Iguchi Y, Grotta JC, Alexandrov AV: Yield and accuracy of urgent combined carotid/transcranial ultrasound testing in acute cerebral ischemia. Stroke 2005;36:32–37.

9 Kasner SE, Chimowitz MI, Lynn MJ, Howlett-Smith H, Stern BJ, Hertzberg VS, Frankel MR, Levine SR, Chaturvedi S, Benesch CG, Sila CA, Jovin TG, Romano JG, Cloft HJ, Warfarin Aspirin Symptomatic Intracranial Disease Trial Investigators: Predictors of ischemic stroke in the territory of a symptomatic intracranial arterial stenosis. Circulation 2006;113: 555–363.

10 Grant EG, Benson CB, Moneta GL, Alexandrov AV, Baker JD, Bluth EI, Carroll BA, Eliasziw M, Gocke J, Hertzberg BS, Katarick S, Needleman L, Pellerito J, Polak JF, Rholl KS, Wooster DL, Zierler E, Society of Radiologists in Ultrasound. Carotid artery stenosis: gray-scale and Doppler US diagnosis – Society of Radiologists in Ultrasound Consensus Conference. Radiology 2003;229:340–346.

11 Goes E, Janssens W, Maillet B, Freson M, Steyaert L, Osteaux M: Tissue characterization of atheromatous plaques: correlation between ultrasound image and histological findings. J Clin Ultrasound 1990;18: 611–613.

12 Barnett HJ, Taylor DW, Eliasziw M, Fox AJ, Ferguson GG, Haynes RB, Rankin RN, Clagett GP, Hachinski VC, Sackett DL, Thorpe KE, Meldrum HE, Spence JD: Benefit of carotid endarterectomy in patients with symptomatic moderate or severe stenosis. North American Symptomatic Carotid Endarterectomy Trial Collaborators. N Engl J Med 1998; 339:1415–1425.

13 Randomised trial of endarterectomy for recently symptomatic carotid stenosis: final results of the MRC European Carotid Surgery Trial (ECST). Lancet 1998;351:1379–1387.

14 Siebler M, Nachtmann A, Sitzer M, Rose G, Kleinschmidt A, Rademacher J, Steinmetz H: Cerebral microembolism and the risk of ischemia in asymptomatic high-grade internal carotid artery stenosis. Stroke 1995;26:2184–186.

15 Gur AY, Bova I, Bornstein NM: Is impaired vasomotor reactivity a predictive factor of stroke in asymptomatic patients? Stroke 1996;27:2188–2190.

16 Spencer MP: Transcranial Doppler monitoring and causes of stroke from carotid endarterectomy. Stroke 1997;28:685–691.

17 Markus HS, Droste DW, Kaps M, Larrue V, Lees KR, Siebler M, Ringelstein EB: Dual antiplatelet therapy with clopidogrel and aspirin in symptomatic carotid stenosis evaluated using Doppler embolic signal detection: The Clopidogrel and Aspirin for Reduction of Emboli in Symptomatic Carotid Stenosis (CARESS) trial. Circulation 2005;111:2233–2240.

18 Spence JD, Tamayo A, Lownie SP, Ng WP, Ferguson GG: Absence of microemboli on transcranial Doppler identifies low-risk patients with asymptomatic carotid stenosis. Stroke 2005;36:2373–2378.

19 Savitz SI, Caplan LR: Vertebrobasilar disease. N Engl J Med 2005;352:2618–2626.

20 Tsivgoulis G, Sharma VK, Hoover SL, Lao AY, Ardelt AA, Malkoff MD, Alexandrov AV: Applications and advantages of power motion-mode Doppler in acute posterior circulation cerebral ischemia. Stroke 2008;39:1197–1204.

21 Saqqur M, Sharma VK, Tsivgoulis G, Huy TN, Heliopoulos I, Siddiqui M, Derksen C, Khan K, Alexandrov AV: Real-time hemodynamic assessment of downstream effects of intracranial stenoses in patients with orthostatic hypoperfusion syndrome. Cerebrovasc Dis 2010;30:355–361.
22 Huang YN, Gao S, Li SW, Huang Y, Li JF, Wong KS, Kay R: Vascular lesions in Chinese patients with transient ischemic attacks. Neurology 1997;48:524–525.
23 Wong KS, Li H, Chan YL, Ahuja A, Lam WW, Wong A, Kay R: Use of transcranial Doppler ultrasound to predict outcome in patients with intracranial large-artery occlusive disease. Stroke 2000;31:2641–2647.
24 Wong KS, Li H: Long-term mortality and recurrent stroke risk among Chinese stroke patients with predominant intracranial atherosclerosis. Stroke 2003;34:2361–2366.
25 Wong KS, Chen C, Fu J, Chang HM, Suwanwela NC, Huang YN, Han Z, Tan KS, Ratanakorn D, Chollate P, Zhao Y, Koh A, Hao Q, Markus HS, CLAIR study investigators: Clopidogrel plus aspirin versus aspirin alone for reducing embolisation in patients with acute symptomatic cerebral or carotid artery stenosis (CLAIR study): a randomised, open-label, blinded-endpoint trial. Lancet Neurol 2010;9:489–497.
26 Messé SR, Silverman IE, Kizer JR, Homma S, Zahn C, Gronseth G, Kasner SE, Quality Standards Subcommittee of the American Academy of Neurology: Practice parameter: recurrent stroke with patent foramen ovale and atrial septal aneurysm: report of the Quality Standards Subcommittee of the American Academy of Neurology. Neurology 2004;62:1042–1050.
27 Lao AY, Sharma VK, Tsivgoulis G, Malkoff MD, Alexandrov AV, Frey JL: Effect of body positioning during transcranial Doppler detection of right-to-left shunts. Eur J Neurol 2007;14:1035–1039.
28 Markus HS, Harrison MJ: Estimation of cerebrovascular reactivity using transcranial Doppler, including the use of breath-holding as the vasodilatory stimulus. Stroke 1992;23:668–673.
29 Alexandrov AV, Sharma VK, Lao AY, Tsivgoulis G, Malkoff MD, Alexandrov AW: Reversed Robin Hood syndrome in acute ischemic stroke patients. Stroke 2007;38:3045–3048.
30 Wojner-Alexander AW, Garami Z, Chernyshev OY, Alexandrov AV: Heads down: flat positioning improves blood flow velocity in acute ischemic stroke. Neurology 2005;64:1354–1357.

Dr. Vijay K. Sharma
Division of Neurology, Department of Medicine
National University Hospital
Singapore 119074 (Singapore)
E-Mail drvijay@singnet.com.sg

Uchiyama S, Amarenco P, Minematsu K, Wong KSL (eds): TIA as Acute Cerebrovascular Syndrome.
Front Neurol Neurosci. Basel, Karger, 2014, vol 33, pp 135–146 (DOI: 10.1159/000351914)

Stroke Subtypes and Interventional Studies for Transient Ischemic Attack

Philippa Lavallée · Pierre Amarenco

INSERM U-698, Department of Neurology and Stroke Center, AP-HP, Bichat-Claude Bernard Hospital, University Paris Diderot, Sorbonne Paris Cité, Paris, France

Abstract

Transient ischemic attack (TIA) is the most important risk factor for ischemic stroke. The risk is the highest in the first hours after symptom onset, and treatment must be initiated in emergency. In the acute phase, antithrombotic agent is probably the most important treatment, but it is not excluded that lipid-lowering agents and/or antihypertensive drugs are also important. For current guidelines, monotherapy of antiplatelet agent remains the gold standard in emergency. However, most recent data and meta-analysis support a combination therapy of clopidogrel and aspirin. Data on treatment in the very acute phase of TIA in the different etiologic stroke subtypes are also lacking especially for cardioembolic stroke and the potential benefit of anticoagulant. Long-term prevention mainly derived from large trials, in which TIA and minor stroke patients have constituted the largest part. Patients with non-cardioembolic stroke must be treated with antiplatelet agent in monotherapy, and dual antiplatelet therapy such as clopidogrel plus aspirin should be avoided, particularly in lacunar strokes, whereas anticoagulants are the treatment of choice for patients with cardioembolic stroke. Major advances concerning stroke prevention in patients with atrial fibrillation have emerged with new oral anticoagulant agents that are as effective as vitamin K antagonists and safer, especially with regard to the risk of intracranial hemorrhage. At variance with moderate and severe cerebral infarction, oral anticoagulants can be initiated without delay in TIA patients. Left atrial appendage closure seems to be a promising treatment in patients ineligible for anticoagulation. Aggressive management of vascular risk factors, including blood pressure as low as 130/80 mm Hg, intensive statin treatment, smoking cessation and diabetes control, also plays a major role in the prevention of vascular event.

As transient ischemic attacks (TIA) and stroke share pathophysiologic mechanisms, causes and risks, principles of secondary prevention are pretty much the same, and most randomized clinical trials of secondary stroke prevention have included TIA either alone or with cerebral infarction with no significant handicap. The main pillars of preventive treatment in TIA patients are identification and treatment of the cause and management of vascular risk factors. Prompt evaluation and adequate treatment have been shown to be highly effective and are the key factors for stroke risk reduction after a TIA [1, 2]. In the present chapter, we will discuss specific management of the main stroke causes (atherosclerosis, atrial fibrillation, AF, and small vessel disease, SVD). General principles for management of vascular risk factors are not within the scope of our topic and will be discussed in dedicated chapters. Acute secondary prevention, independent of stroke subtype, will also be shortly discussed.

The etiological classification of ischemic stroke has been defined as large artery atherosclerotic (LAA) disease, which may be extracranial or intracranial; embolism from a cardiac source; SVD; other determined cause (e.g. dissection, hypercoagulable states, vasculitis), and infarcts of undetermined cause [3]. Whatever the cause of cerebral infarction, treatment still relies on the use of antithrombotic. We will see that the choice of antithrombotic depends on stroke subtypes but that in some cases further treatment is necessary.

Acute Management of Patients with Transient Ischemic Attack Independently of Stroke Subtype

Prospective studies have shown that stroke risk is high after a TIA: 3.1% (95% CI: 2.0–4.1) at 2 days and 5.2% (3.9–6.5) at 7 days [4]. Secondary prevention should be initiated as soon as possible, as early and intensive management (antithrombotic agent, vascular factor management, revascularization procedure if necessary) of these patients in a dedicated clinic has shown efficacy in reducing the risk of stroke by 80% in 2 studies [1, 2]. In both studies, specific details such as delay or type of antithrombotic drugs, exact delay for administration of statin or lowering blood pressure therapy are lacking. So, no conclusion concerning the relative contributions of the different aspects of their treatment to the benefit observed can be drawn. The FASTER (Fast Assessment of Stroke and Transient Ischemic Attack to prevent Early Recurrence) pilot trial [5], is the first trial dedicated to the treatment of patients in the very acute phase of minor stroke and TIA. There was no stroke subtype restriction. Patients were randomly assigned within 24 h to clopidogrel or its placebo on top of aspirin, and were separately randomly assigned to simvastatin or its placebo. The primary outcome was stroke (ischemic and hemorrhagic) at 90 days. Safety outcomes included hemorrhage related to clopidogrel and myositis related to simvastatin. Unfortunately, the study was stopped prematurely due to failure of recruitment. The risk of stroke was nonsignificantly decreased in the clopidogrel plus aspirin group in comparison with the aspirin group [7.1 vs. 10.8%, risk ratio 0.7 (95% CI: 0.3–1.2)]. Two patients on clopidogrel had intracranial hemorrhage compared with none on the placebo [absolute risk increase 1.0% (–0.4 to 2.4); p = 0.5]. No benefit was observed in the simvastatin group. Data are still too limited to recommend the combination of aspirin and clopidogrel in the acute phase of TIA. However the result of three large trials (CHANCE [6],

POINT and TARDIS) testing combination of antiplatelet agents in the very acute phase of TIA or minor score are coming and could change daily practice. The results of the CHANCE trial have been recently presented at the last International Stroke Conference. 5,170 Chinese patients were randomly assigned within 24 h of symptom onset to clopidogrel (300-mg loading dose followed by 75 mg daily) plus aspirin 75 mg for the first 21 days followed by clopidogrel until 90 days or to aspirin alone. The primary outcome (ischemic and hemorrhagic stroke within the first 90 days) occurred in 11.7% of the aspirin alone group compared with 8.2% of the clopidogrel plus aspirin group (hazard ratio, HR = 0.68; 95% CI: 0.57–0.81). The risk of hemorrhagic stroke was very small (0.3%) and similar in both groups.

Data on anticoagulant therapy in the acute phase of TIA are lacking. No data are available concerning blood pressure-lowering therapy or lipid-lowering agent (except in the FASTER trial [5]) in this population. Moreover, secondary prevention trials considering stroke subtypes in the acute phase of TIA do not exist, limiting the generalization of the available results.

Large Artery Atherosclerotic Disease

LAA is directly responsible for about 30% of TIAs. However, in 90% of cases, investigations find some form of atherosclerotic disease (regardless of the degree of stenosis) in intra- or extracranial arteries or in the thoracic aorta of coronary arteries. Importantly, the main large secondary stroke prevention trials that have tested antiplatelet agents [7–9] have also included patients with other non-cardioembolic stroke such as patients with SVD or with undetermined causes (stroke of presumed arterial origin).

Antithrombotic Regimen

Antiplatelet therapy has proven to be effective in reducing major vascular events (non-fatal myocardial infarction, non-fatal stroke, or vascular death) among patients with non-cardioembolic stroke or TIA. On average, antiplatelet agents reduce the risk of major vascular events by about 22% and should be administered as soon as possible after TIA [10]. Several antiplatelet drugs are available: aspirin, combination aspirin/dipyridamole, clopidogrel, ticlopidine, cilostazol and triflusal (not all of them have been approved by all drugs agencies). All of these agents are effective in major vascular event prevention after a TIA.

The choice depends on efficacy, tolerance, patient profile, price and availability. Aspirin is by far the cheapest drug. The combination of aspirin/dipyridamole is more effective than aspirin alone to prevent major vascular event or major bleeding, but tolerance such as headaches and bleeding could limit its clinical value [11, 12]. The combination of aspirin/dipyridamole has also been compared with clopidogrel alone and failed to show non-inferiority for recurrent stroke or major vascular event occurrence [13]. In this study, the combination therapy was associated with more major hemorrhagic events including intracranial hemorrhage even though the net benefit with regard to the risk of recurrent stroke or major hemorrhagic event was similar in the two groups. Compared to aspirin, clopidogrel achieved a nonsignificant reduction of major vascular events with similar safety profile [14]. Because of safety concern, the use of ticlopidine is now limited in daily clinical practice [15]. Triflusal, which has not been approved by all drug agencies, has similar efficacy than aspirin for secondary prevention of serious vascular events and was associated with a lower risk of hemorrhagic complications [16].

In conclusion, aspirin (75–150 mg/day), the combination of aspirin (38–300 mg/day) and dipyridamole (200 mg extended release twice daily), clopidogrel (75 mg/day) or triflusal (600 mg/day) are all good options in first-line therapy for prevention of major vascular events in patient with TIA from arterial origin.

There is also some evidence that a short course of dual antiplatelet treatment could be effective in the prevention of major vascular events in the very acute period after a TIA or minor stroke especially for those related to LAA. The MATCH [17], CHARISMA [18] and FASTER [5] studies, which have compared in patients with non-cardioembolic stroke, the effectiveness of aspirin plus clopidogrel with, respectively, clopidogrel alone or aspirin alone, showed a trend in favor of the combination therapy in patients included in the acute setting. Microembolic signals are common in patients with LAA and are an independent marker of future stroke risk in patients with extracranial disease [19] or intracranial stenosis [20]. In the CARESS [21] and CLAIR [22] studies, dual therapy with clopidogrel and aspirin was more effective than aspirin alone in reducing microembolic signals in the acute phase of stroke or TIA related to intracranial and extracranial LAA. To date, these data are still too limited to recommend the combination of aspirin and clopidogrel in the acute setting of TIA due to LAA or to presume arterial origin. Recently, the CHANCE trial performed in 5,000 Chinese stroke patients found at 90 days a 32% reduction in new ischemic or hemorrhagic stroke with no increase in major hemorrhages when dual antiplatelet therapy was compared with aspirin alone during 21 days, followed by monotherapy of clopidogrel versus aspirin until 90 days [6]. One other exception could be TIA due to high grade intracranial atherosclerosis since a short course of clopidogrel plus aspirin on top of intensive management of vascular risk factors was associated with an unexpected low rate of stroke recurrence in the SAMMPRIS trial (see below) [23].

Revascularization Procedures

Extracranial Carotid Artery Disease

Carotid endarterectomy is the gold standard for stroke prevention in patients with severe symptomatic internal carotid stenosis. Pooled analysis of data from randomized controlled trials indicates that carotid endarterectomy significantly reduces risk of stroke in patients with 50% or greater stenosis who have had a TIA or previous non-disabling stroke. Surgery was highly beneficial in patients with 70–99% stenosis and moderate in patients with 50–69% stenosis with a significant absolute risk reduction of ipsilateral ischemic stroke of 16 and 4.6%, respectively. Surgery was ineffective or even harmful in patients with carotid near occlusion or carotid stenosis of <50% [24]. Carotid endarterectomy should be performed as soon as possible as benefits of surgery quickly diminish after 14 days of symptom onset [25]. Carotid endarterectomy should only be performed in expert centers with a perioperative complication rate (all strokes and death) of <6% for patients with >70% stenosis and <3% for patients with 50–69% stenosis.

Carotid angioplasty and stenting (CAS) has emerged as a therapeutic alternative to carotid endarterectomy for treatment of severe extracranial carotid stenosis. The proposed advantages of CAS are its less invasive nature, decreasing the risk of cranial nerve palsy and patient discomfort. A meta-analysis of 4 randomized trials including patients with a recent symptomatic severe carotid stenosis compared the two strategies and indicated that patients who received CAS had a significant increased risk of 30-day death or stroke compared with patients who received carotid endarterectomy (odds ratio 1.60; 95% CI: 1.26–2.02) related to periprocedural complications of CAS [26]. After the periprocedural period, the risk of ipsilateral stroke was low and similar in both treatment groups, suggesting that the safety of carotid stenting needs to be improved before it can be used as an alternative to carotid endarterectomy in patients with symptomatic carotid stenosis. However, the CREST trial [27] and the meta-analysis of the 3 European trials has suggested that in patients younger than 70 years, stenting procedure could be a fair alternative to surgery [28].

In conclusion, TIA patients with symptomatic high-grade extracranial carotid stenosis (especially those with >70% stenosis) should undergo carotid endarterectomy as soon as possible (and definitely within 14 days) by expert surgeons. Stenting should be restricted to selected high-risk patients (e.g. those with contraindications to CEA, stenosis at a surgically inaccessible site, re-stenosis after earlier CEA, and post-radiation stenosis) and, in experienced centers, to patients younger than 70 years.

Intracranial Artery Disease

Symptomatic intracranial stenosis confers a very high risk of stroke recurrence despite the use of antithrombotic treatment such as aspirin or anticoagulant [29]. The surgical option with extracranial-intracranial bypass procedures was abandoned due to the lack of benefit over medical therapy in patients with middle cerebral artery disease [30]. Recently, the SAMMPRIS trial showed that aggressive medical management alone was superior to intracranial arterial stenting in addition to aggressive medical therapy in patients with a recent TIA or stroke attributed to severe stenosis of a major intracranial artery [23]. Despite negative result for the stenting hypothesis, the SAMMPRIS study has important positive implications as it has shown that aggressive medical management (target systolic blood pressure factor <140 mm Hg; LDL cholesterol level <0.70 g/l; clopidogrel in addition to aspirin for the 90 days after enrollment) dramatically decreased the risk of stroke or death. The one-year risk of stroke and death in the aggressive medical management arm of the SAMMPRIS trial was

12.2% in comparison with 25% in patients with aspirin or coumadin in the previously published WASID study.

In conclusion, revascularization procedures are not recommended for TIA patients with symptomatic intracranial stenosis related to atherosclerosis until another trial shows positive results. In the meantime, aggressive management of vascular risk factors and a short course of aspirin plus clopidogrel seem to be a very effective therapy.

Small Vessel Disease

SVD accounts for about 20% of TIA; despite high prevalence, few large prevention trials have been dedicated to these patients.

Two very large trials have established the role antiplatelet therapy in the acute phase of stroke, and in each, their effect on the lacunar stroke subtype has been reported [31, 32] and was similar to those found on stroke due to atherosclerosis. In the prospectively planned meta-analysis of the two studies, early aspirin statistically significantly reduced, by 7 per 1,000, the risk of having a recurrent ischemic stroke within 14–28 days. This occurred in 1.6% of aspirin users versus 2.3% on placebo. There was a trend towards an increase of 2 per 1,000 in the risk of having a hemorrhagic stroke or hemorrhagic transformation. The overall risk reduction of any further death of stroke was of 9 per 1,000 [33].

Until recently, data on long-term vascular prevention in patients with SVD were scarce, as no large clinical trials had been dedicated to these patients, although they accounted for more than 50% in the CAPRIE [14], MATCH [17] and PRoFESS [13] trials. Hence, it is assumed that the benefit of antiplatelet agents in terms of major vascular event risk reduction observed in patients with non-cardioembolic stroke can be generalizable to patients with SVD. Subgroup analysis of large randomized trials emphasized this assumption. In the CATS trial [34], ticlopidine 250 mg twice daily was associated with a relative reduction of recurrent stroke, myocardial infarction and death of 30% in comparison to placebo in patients with stroke due to LAA and SVD with no significant difference between the two groups. In the AICLA trial [35], aspirin and the combination of aspirin and dipyridamole reduced the relative risk of stroke recurrence by 70% in comparison with placebo in patients with SVD. There was no difference between aspirin and the combination therapy, but the sample size was small. In the CSPS study, cilostazol was found to reduce the risk of secondary stroke by 41.7% compared with placebo. A risk reduction of 43% was observed in patients with SVD (which accounted for 75% of the cohort) [36].

The SPS3 trial is the first large secondary prevention trial dedicated to patients with SVD. Patients with a recent symptomatic stroke related to SVD were randomized in a two-by-two factorial design: clopidogrel and aspirin versus aspirin alone and two target levels of systolic blood pressure. The antiplatelet part of the trial was terminated prematurely on the recommendation of the data and safety monitoring committee.

Compared to aspirin alone, the combination of aspirin and clopidogrel did not decrease the risk of recurrent stroke (2.7 vs. 2.5%/year, respectively) but almost doubled the risk of brain hemorrhage (1.1 vs. 2.1%/year) [37]. The blood pressure part of the study has not been published yet.

In conclusion, after a TIA due to SVD, antiplatelet agent (aspirin, clopidogrel, cilostazol, or the combination of aspirin and dipyridamole) should be initiated as soon as possible. Dual therapy with clopidogrel and aspirin is no better than monotherapy in these patients.

Atrial Fibrillation

AF accounts for 10–12% of ischemic strokes and is associated with a very high risk of stroke recurrence (about 12%/year). The European Atrial Fibrillation Trial assessed the effects of antithrombotic treatment in patients who had a recent TIA or ischemic stroke due to AF [38]. This study showed that in comparison to placebo, vitamin K antagonists (VKAs) with an INR 2.5–4.0 dramatically decreased the risk of vascular death, myocardial infarction, stroke, or systemic emboli (HR 0.53, 0.36–0.79), with no increase in major hemorrhages in that study. A meta-analysis [39] established VKAs with a target INR 2.5 (2–3) as the gold standard for antithrombotic treatment of patients with TIA or stroke and AF. In daily practice, concerns about the increased risk of intracranial hemorrhages and the need for careful monitoring of treatment lead to underuse of warfarin. In the last years, major efforts have been made to find alternative solutions with positive results.

Recently, 4 major trials have studied new anticoagulant agents, a direct thrombin inhibitor (dabigatran) and three direct factor Xa inhibitors (rivaroxaban, apixaban and edoxaban), in patients with AF at low, moderate or high risk of stroke. Pre-specified subgroup analyses of subjects with prior TIA or stroke have been published for the 3 first drugs. The RE-LY trial [40] compared open-label warfarin with 2 fixed doses of dabigatran (110 or 150 mg twice daily). For patients with previous TIA or stroke, the rate of stroke or systemic embolism was not statistically different with warfarin (2.78% per year), dabigatran 150 (2.07% per year) or dabigatran 110 (2.32% per year). The rate of major bleeding was significantly lower in patients on dabigatran 110 mg/day and similar in those on dabigatran 150 mg/day compared with those on warfarin. The rate of intracranial bleeding was lower for either dose of dabigatran in comparison to warfarin. The ROCKET-AF trial [41] was a double-blind non-inferiority trial that randomized non-valvular AF patients at moderate or high risk of stroke to rivaroxaban (20 mg/day) or dose-adjusted warfarin (target INR: 2.0–3.0). Among subjects with a history of prior stroke, TIA, or systemic embolism, the primary efficacy end point (composite of ischemic and hemorrhagic stroke or systemic embolism) was similar in both groups [4.8% in the rivaroxaban group vs. 4.9% in the warfarin group (HR, 0.98; 95% CI: 0.8–1.2)], as well as the primary safety end point [a composite of major and non-major clinically relevant bleeding; 3.5% with rivaroxaban vs. 3.9% with warfarin (HR, 0.91; 95% CI: 0.72–1.14)]. The ARISTOTLE trial [42] was a double-blind, randomized trial comparing apixaban (5 mg twice daily or 2.5 mg twice daily if patients met two or more of the following criteria: age ≥80 years, body weight ≤60 kg, or serum creatinine ≥1.5 mg/dl) with warfarin (target INR: 2.0–3.0) for the prevention of stroke (ischemic or hemorrhagic) or systemic embolism among patients with AF or flutter and at least 1 additional risk factor for stroke. In the subgroup of patients with previous stroke or TIA, the rate of stroke or systemic embolism was 2.46 per 100 patient-years of follow-up in the apixaban group and 3.24 in the warfarin group (HR, 0.76; 95% CI: 0.56–1.03). The reduction in the primary outcome of stroke or systemic embolism was mainly driven by a reduction in hemorrhagic stroke. The absolute reduction in hemorrhagic stroke with apixaban compared with warfarin was 0.60% per year in patients with previous stroke. If there is no doubt that new oral anticoagulation agents represent a good alternative to VKAs for stroke prevention in patients with AF, limitations remain such as previous major hemorrhage, severe renal impairment, very old people but also cost.

Conversely, it has been shown that the association of aspirin and clopidogrel is less effective than VKAs and should not be used in patients eligible to oral anticoagulation [43].

The best way to avoid hemorrhage is to avoid antithrombotic treatment. In AF, more than 90% of atrial thrombus originates from the left atrial appendage. It has been hypothesized that the isolation of left atrial appendage from the systemic circulation should reduce the risk of stroke and other systemic embolism. The PROTECT-AF study is a multicenter, non-inferiority trial, which has tested the non-inferiority of the combination of percutaneous left atrial appendage closure device (WATCHMAN) and short-term (3 months) warfarin as compared with long-term warfarin therapy alone in patients with AF and a CHADS2 score of 1 or more [44]. The probability of non-inferiority of the device was more than 99.9% with regard to the primary efficacy end point (occurrence of all types of stroke, cardiovascular or unexplained death, or systemic emboli within up to 3 years), and patients who received the device had fewer hemorrhagic strokes than the controls. However, the primary safety end point (which combined major bleeding, serious pericardial effusion, and device embolization) was significantly greater in the device group than in the control group (relative increase of 1.69, 95% Bayesian credible interval 1.01–3.19), mostly due to 22 (4.8%) patients undergoing drainage of serious pericardial effusions. Despite promising results, this study had two main limitations: most of the patients had CHADS2 scores of 1 or 2 (explaining the low rate of stroke observed in both groups) and the mean age of the patients (just above 70 years) was rather low compared with daily practice. For now, the WATCHMAN device is probably best applied in patients with AF at high risk of stroke ineligible for anticoagulant therapy and those who have experienced stroke despite anticoagulation therapy. Further studies are required to confirm this hypothesis.

For patients ineligible for VKA treatment, several options could be chosen depending on the type of contraindications. In the case of inability (confirmed or supposed) to maintain an INR within the therapeutic range or if INR could not be assessed at requested intervals, apixaban (5 mg twice daily or 2.5 mg twice daily if patients met two or more of the following criteria: age ≥80 years, body weight ≤60 kg, or serum creatinine ≥1.5 mg/dl) is probably the best option over aspirin therapy. In the AVERROES trial in which patients unsuitable for VKA treatment, but with no contraindication to anticoagulation, were randomly assigned to apixaban versus aspirin, those allocated to apixaban had fewer primary outcome events (RR 0.45, 0.32–0.62), and no excess of major hemorrhages [45]. In the case of contraindication to anticoagulation because of an increased risk of hemorrhage, left atrial appendage closure could possibly be an option, but long-term randomized trials are lacking, especially in old patients [44]. Aspirin (75–100 mg/day) has little effect in this indication but is more effective than placebo, with an estimated relative risk reduction of 21% [46]. It is a reasonable alternative in patients with contraindications to anticoagulation if left atrial appendage closure is not possible. The combination therapy of aspirin and clopidogrel versus aspirin alone in patients with AF and moderate or high risk of stroke who were not eligible for VKAs slightly decrease the risk of ischemic events (RR 0.89, 0.81–0.98), but this benefit was counterbalanced by an increased risk of bleeding complications (1.57, 1.29–1.92) [47]. However, the European Society of Cardiology guidelines recommend dual antiplatelet therapy over aspirin alone based on the ACTIVE-A TRIAL in the case of ineligibility for oral anticoagulant (although the ACTIVE-A trial showed increased risk of major hemorrhage in the clopidogrel plus aspirin group).

In conclusion, for patients with TIA and AF and no contraindication to anticoagulation, VKAs or new anticoagulant agents (apixaban 5 mg twice a day, dabigatran 150 mg twice a day and rivaroxaban 2 mg/day) are all good options. New anticoagulant agents have immense advantages over VKAs, and the European Society of Cardiology guidelines recommend these agents over VKAs in most cases. They are also contraindicated in the case of severe renal insufficiency (creatinine clearance <30 ml/min for rivaroxaban and dabigatran, <25 ml/min for apixaban). Because of an increased risk of hemorrhage, the dose of dabigatran should be reduced to 110 mg twice a day in certain cases, mainly moderate renal insufficiency (creatinine clearance 30–50 ml/min), older patients (>75 or 80 years), gastritis or esophagitis and low-weight patients (<50 kg). The dose of rivaroxaban should be reduced to 15 mg/day in the case of moderate renal insufficiency (creatinine clearance 15–49 ml/min). The dose of apixaban should be reduced to 2.5 mg/day if patients meet two or more of the following criteria: age ≥80 years, body weight ≤60 kg, or serum creatinine ≥1.5 mg/dl. Careful information should be given to patients and their families about the importance of compliance. Because of the short half-life of these medications, patients who are noncompliant and miss medication doses might be at risk for thromboembolism.

For patients with TIA and AF and unsuitable for VKAs but not for anticoagulation, apixaban is the best treatment option.

For patients with TIA and AF and unsuitable for anticoagulation, left atrial appendage closure is a possible alternative strategy in combination with a 3-month course of VKA, but more trials are needed to establish this procedure. Aspirin has no proven effect except in a meta-analysis.

The optimal delay to start anticoagulation after a TIA and AF is unknown. These patients are at higher risk of stroke in comparison to patients with TIA due to SVD or of unknown cause [48]. If in the first 2 weeks of an ischemic stroke, the risk of hemorrhagic transformation of a fresh brain infarct seems to offset any benefits from reduction of recurrent embolic ischemic stroke, this is unlikely to be the case for TIA or small ischemic stroke [49]. This question has not been formally addressed in patients with TIA, but starting immediate anticoagulation is reasonable, and probably safe in this setting.

Conclusion

Preventive treatment in the acute phase of TIA is very efficient in the prevention of stroke recurrence and should be started as soon as possible. Treatment is mainly based on antithrombotic drugs, management of vascular risk factor and endarterectomy/ stenting in the case of high-grade carotid stenosis. If long-term prevention is now well established, further studies are required for the acute setting where the risk of stroke is particularly high. Answers are lacking concerning the choice of antithrombotic agent (one antiplatelet agent versus dual, triple antiplatelet agents or anticoagulant), the need of emergent blood pressure-lowering therapy and/or lipid-lowering agent. It would be also important to know if preventive treatment should be tailored to stroke subtypes.

References

1 Lavallee PC, Meseguer E, Abboud H, et al: A transient ischaemic attack clinic with round-the-clock access (SOS-TIA): feasibility and effects. Lancet Neurol 2007;6:953–960.

2 Rothwell PM, Giles MF, Chandratheva A, et al, on behalf of the Early use of Existing Preventive Strategies for Stroke (EXPRESS) study. Effect of urgent treatment of transient ischaemic attack and minor stroke on early recurrent stroke (EXPRESS study): a prospective population-based sequential comparison. Lancet 2007;370:1432–1442.

3 Amarenco P, Bogousslavsky J, Caplan LR, Donnan GA, Hennerici MG: New approach to stroke subtyping: the A-S-C-O (phenotypic) classification of stroke. Cerebrovasc Dis 2009;27:502–508.

4 Giles MF, Rothwell PM: Risk of stroke early after transient ischaemic attack: a systematic review and meta-analysis. Lancet Neurol 2007;6:1063–1072.

5 Kennedy J, Hill MD, Ryckborst KJ, et al, for the FASTER Investigators: Fast assessment of stroke and transient ischaemic attack to prevent early recurrence (FASTER): a randomised controlled pilot trial. Lancet Neurol 2007;6:961–969.

6 Wang Y, Johnston SC, CHANCE investigators: Rationale and design of a randomized, double-blind trial comparing the effects of a 3-month clopidogrel-aspirin regimen versus aspirin alone for the treatment of high-risk patients with acute nondisabling cerebrovascular event. Am Heart J 2010;160:380–386.

7 UK-TIA Study Group: The United Kingdom Transient Ischaemic Attack (UK-TIA) aspirin trial: final results. J Neurol Neurosurg Psychiatry 1991;54:1044–1054.

8 The Dutch TIA Trial Study Group: A comparison of two doses of aspirin (30 vs. 283 mg a day) in patients after a transient ischemic attack or minor ischemic stroke. N Engl J Med 1991;325:1261–1266.
9 The SALT Collaborative Group. Swedish Aspirin Low-dose Trial (SALT) of 75 mg aspirin as secondary prophylaxis after cerebrovascular ischaemic events. Lancet 1991;338:1345–1349.
10 Antiplatelet Trialists' Collaboration: Collaborative overview of randomised trials of antiplatelet therapy. I. prevention of death, myocardial infarction, and stroke by prolonged antiplatelet therapy in various categories of patients. BMJ 1994;308:81–106.
11 Diener HC, Cunha L, Forbes C, Sivenius J, Smets P, Lowenthal A: European Stroke Prevention Study. 2. Dipyridamole and acetylsalicylic acid in the secondary prevention of stroke. J Neurol Sci 1996;143: 1–13.
12 The ESPRIT Study Group: Aspirin plus dipyridamole versus aspirin alone after cerebral ischaemia of arterial origin (ESPRIT): randomised controlled trial. Lancet 2006;367:1665–1673.
13 Sacco RL, Diener H-C, Yusuf S, Cotton D, Ounpuu S, Lawton WA, Palesch Y, Martin RH, Albers GW, Bath P, Bornstein N, Chan BP, Chen ST, Cunha L, Dahlöf B, De Keyser J, Donnan GA, Estol C, Gorelick P, Gu V, Hermansson K, Hilbrich L, Kaste M, Lu C, Machnig T, Pais P, Roberts R, Skvortsova V, Teal P, Toni D, Vandermaelen C, Voigt T, Weber M, Yoon BW, PRoFESS Study Group: Aspirin and extended-release dipyridamole versus clopidogrel for recurrent stroke. N Engl J Med 2008;359:1238–1251.
14 CAPRIE Steering Committee: A randomised, blinded, trial of clopidogrel versus aspirin in patients at risk of ischaemic events (CAPRIE). Lancet 1996;348: 1329–1339.
15 Hass WK, Easton JD, Adams HP, Pryse-Phillips W, Molony BA, Anderson S, Kamm B, the Ticlopidine Aspirin Stroke Study Group: A randomized trial comparing ticlopidine hydrochloride with aspirin for the prevention of stroke in high-risk patients. N Engl J Med 1989;321:501–507.
16 Matias-Guiu J, Ferro JM, Alvarez-Sabin J, Calvo G, the TACIP Study Group: Triflusal versus aspirin in secondary stroke prevention: results of TACIP Study. Stroke 2003;34:840–848.
17 Diener HC, Bogousslavsky J, Brass LM, et al, the MATCH investigators. Aspirin and clopidogrel compared with clopidogrel alone after recent ischaemic stroke or transient ischaemic attack in high-risk patients (MATCH): randomised, double-blind, placebo-controlled trial. Lancet 2004;364:331–337.
18 Hankey GJ, Johnston SC, Easton JD, et al, CHARISMA trial investigators: Effect of clopidogrel plus ASA vs ASA early after TIA and ischaemic stroke: a substudy of the CHARISMA trial. Int J Stroke 2011;6:3–9.
19 Markus HS, MacKinnon A: Asymptomatic embolization detected by Doppler ultrasound predicts stroke risk in symptomatic carotid artery stenosis. Stroke 2005;36:971–975.
20 Gao S, Wong KS, Hansberg T, Lam WW, Droste DW, Ringelstein EB: Microembolic signal predicts recurrent cerebral ischemic events in acute stroke patients with middle cerebral artery stenosis. Stroke 2004;35:2832–2836.
21 Markus HS, Droste DW, Kaps M, et al: Dual antiplatelet therapy with clopidogrel and aspirin in symptomatic carotid stenosis evaluated using Doppler embolic detection signal detection: the Clopidogrel and Aspirin for Reduction of Emboli in Symptomatic Carotid Stenosis (CARESS) trial. Circulation 2005;111:2233–2240.
22 Wong KSL, Chen C, Fu J, et al, the CLAIR study investigators: Clopidogrel plus aspirin versus aspirin alone for reducing embolisation in patients with acute symptomatic cerebral or carotid artery stenosis (CLAIR study): a randomised, open-label, blinded-endpoint trial. Lancet Neurol 2010;9:489–497.
23 Chimowitz MI, Lynn MJ, Derdeyn CP, et al: Stenting versus aggressive medical therapy for intracranial arterial stenosis. N Engl J Med 2011;365:993–1003.
24 Rothwell PM, Eliasziw M, Gutnikov SA, Fox AJ, Taylor DW, Mayberg MR, Warlow CP, Barnett HJM, the Carotid Endarterectomy Trialists' Collaboration: Analysis of pooled data from the randomised controlled trials of endarterectomy for symptomatic carotid stenosis. Lancet 2003;361:107–116.
25 Rothwell PM, Eliasziw M, Gutnikov SA, Warlow CP, Barnett HJM, the Carotid Endarterectomy Trialists' Collaboration. Endarterectomy for symptomatic carotid stenosis in relation to clinical subgroups and timing of surgery. Lancet 2004;363:915–924.
26 Amarenco P, Labreuche J, Mazighi M: Lessons from carotid endarterectomy and stenting trials. Lancet 2010;376:1028–1031.
27 Brott TG, Hobson RW, Howard G, Roubin GS, Clark WN, Brooks W, Mackey A, Hill MD, Leimgruber PP, Sheffet AJ, Howard VJ, Moore WS, Voeks JH, Hopkins LN, Cutlip DE, Cohen DJ, Popma JJ, Ferguson RD, Cohen SN, Blackshear JL, Silver FL, Mohr JP, Lal BK, Meschia JF, the CREST Investigators: Stenting versus endarterectomy for treatment of carotid-artery stenosis. N Engl J Med 2010;363:11–23.
28 Carotid Stenting Trialists' Collaboration: Short-term outcome after stenting versus endarterectomy for symptomatic carotid stenosis: a preplanned meta-analysis of individual patient data. Lancet 2010;376: 1062–1073.
29 Chimowitz MI, Lynn MJ, Howlett-Smith H, et al: Comparison of warfarin and aspirin for symptomatic intracranial arterial stenosis. N Engl J Med 2005; 352:1305–1316.

30 The EC/IC Bypass Study Group: Failure of extracranial-intracranial arterial bypass to reduce the risk of ischemic stroke: results of an international randomized trial. N Engl J Med 1985;313:1191–1200.

31 CAST (Chinese Acute Stroke Trial) Collaborative Group: CAST: a randomised placebo-controlled trial of early aspirin use in 20,000 patients with acute ischaemic stroke. Lancet 1997;349:1641–1649.

32 International Stroke Trial Collaborative Group: The International Stroke Trial (IST): a randomised trial of aspirin, subcutaneous heparin, both, or neither among 19,435 patients with acute ischaemic stroke. Lancet 1997;349:1569–1581.

33 Chen ZM, Sandercock S, Pan HC, Counsell C, Collins R, Liu LS, Xie JX, Warlow C, Peto R: Indications for early aspirin use in acute ischemic stroke: a combined analysis of 40,000 randomized patients from the Chinese Acute Stroke Trial and the International Stroke Trial. Stroke 2000;31:1240–1249.

34 Gent M, Easton JD, Hachinski VC, Panak E, Sicurella J, Blakely JA, Ellis DJ, Harbison JW, Roberts RS, Turpie AGG: The Canadian American Ticlopidine Study (CATS) in Thromboembolic Stroke. Lancet 1989;i:1215–1220.

35 Bousser MG, Eschwege E, Haguenau M, Lefauconnier JM, Thibult N, Touboul D, Touboul PJ: 'AICLA' controlled trial of aspirin and dipyridamole in the secondary prevention of athero-thrombotic cerebral ischemia. Stroke 1983;14:5–14.

36 Gotoh F, Tohgi H, Hiraietal S, et al: Cilostazol stroke prevention study: a placebo-controlled double-blind trial for secondary prevention of cerebral infarction. J Stroke Cerebrovasc Dis 2000;9:147–157.

37 The SPS3 Investigators: Effects of clopidogrel added to aspirin in patients with recent lacunar stroke. N Engl J Med 2012;367:817–825.

38 EAFT (European Atrial Fibrillation Trial) Study Group: Secondary prevention in non-rheumatic atrial fibrillation after transient ischaemic attack or minor stroke. Lancet 1993;342:1255–1262.

39 Hart RG, Pearce LA, Aguilar MI: Meta-analysis: antithrombotic therapy to prevent stroke in patients who have nonvalvular atrial fibrillation. Ann Intern Med 2007;146:857–867.

40 Diener H-C, Connolly SJ, Ezekowitz MD, et al, the RE-LY study group: Dabigatran compared with warfarin in patients with atrial fibrillation and previous transient ischaemic attack or stroke: a subgroup analysis of the RE-LY trial. Lancet Neurol 2010;9: 1157–1163.

41 Hankey GJ, Patel MR, Stevens SR, et al, the ROCKET AF Steering Committee Investigators: Rivaroxaban compared with warfarin in patients with atrial fibrillation and previous stroke or transient ischaemic attack: a subgroup analysis of ROCKET AF. Lancet Neurol 2012;11:315–322.

42 Easton JD, Lopes RD, Bahit MC, et al, for the ARISTOTLE Committees and Investigators: Apixaban compared with warfarin in patients with atrial fibrillation and previous stroke or transient ischaemic attack: a subgroup analysis of the ARISTOTLE trial. Lancet Neurol 2012;11:503–511.

43 The ACTIVE Writing Group on behalf of the ACTIVE Investigators: Clopidogrel plus aspirin versus oral anticoagulation for atrial fibrillation in the Atrial fibrillation Clopidogrel Trial with Irbesartan for prevention of Vascular Events (ACTIVE W): a randomised controlled trial. Lancet 2006;367:1903–1912.

44 Holmes DR, Reddy VY, Turi ZG, Doshi SK, Sievert H, Buchbinder M, Mullin CM, Sick P: Percutaneous closure of the left atrial appendage versus warfarin therapy for prevention of stroke in patients with atrial fibrillation: a randomised non-inferiority trial. Lancet 2009;374:534–542.

45 Connolly S, Eikelboom J, Joyner C, Diener C, Hart R, Golitsyn S, et al: Apixaban in patients with atrial fibrillation. N Engl J Med 2011;364:806–817.

46 Singer DE, Albers GW, Dalen JE, Fang MC, Go AS, Halperin JL, Lip GY, Manning WJ: Antithrombotic therapy in atrial fibrillation: American College of Chest Physicians Evidence-Based Clinical Practice Guidelines, ed 8. Chest 2008;133(suppl 6):546S–592S.

47 The ACTIVE Investigators: Effect of clopidogrel added to aspirin in patients with atrial fibrillation. N Engl J Med 2009;360:2066–2067

48 Purroy F, Montaner J, Molina CA, Delgado P, Ribo M, Álvarez-Sabín MJ: Patterns and predictors of early risk of recurrence after transient ischemic attack with respect to etiologic subtypes. Stroke 2007;38: 3225–3229.

49 Paciaroni M, Agnelli G, Micheli S, Caso V: Efficacy and safety of anticoagulant treatment in acute cardioembolic stroke: a meta-analysis of randomized controlled trials. Stroke 2007;38:423–430.

Prof. Pierre Amarenco
Department of Neurology and Stroke Centre, AP-HP, Bichat-Claude Bernard Hospital
University Paris Diderot, Sorbonne Paris Cité, INSERM U698
46, rue Henri Huchard, FR–75018 Paris (France)
E-Mail pierre.amarenco@bch.aphp.fr

Uchiyama S, Amarenco P, Minematsu K, Wong KSL (eds): TIA as Acute Cerebrovascular Syndrome.
Front Neurol Neurosci. Basel, Karger, 2014, vol 33, pp 147–161 (DOI: 10.1159/000351915)

Antithrombotic Therapy in Transient Ischemic Attack Patients

V.E. Held · M.E. Wolf · M.G. Hennerici

Department of Neurology, UniversitätsMedizin Mannheim, University of Heidelberg, Mannheim, Germany

Abstract

Historically, studies of antithrombotic therapy in ischemic cerebrovascular disease have included both stroke and transient ischemic attack (TIA). Thus, therapy regimes are very similar. Aspirin (75–325 mg within 48 h after onset of symptoms) is still the standard antithrombotic treatment because other agents have performed similarly (or worse). Combinations of agents have shown mixed results. Aspirin combined with clopidogrel has failed to show a significant reduction of stroke/TIA recurrences but increased the bleeding risk if taken for more than several months. The combination of aspirin and dipyridamole is slightly better than aspirin alone and in particular reduced nonfatal stroke/TIA – hence it is recommended as an alternative and may be used in patients with recurrent events while on regular aspirin. In contrast, combined treatment is regularly recommended after endovascular interventions and if both cardio- and cerebrovascular diseases are present. Warfarin and similar compounds have long been the standard treatment for most patients with permanent, paroxysmal or intermittent non-valvular atrial fibrillation, for which there is excellent evidence in most patients (CHADS-VASc score >1). New compounds have been approved in recent years and shown to reduce either ischemic events, intracranial bleeding complications or both when compared with warfarin. None of them requires regular therapy monitoring. Because there are no head-to-head comparisons of these newer agents, definite recommendations as to which to choose, and when, are hard to make. However, there are some notable differences as well as new approved entities.

Antiplatelet Therapy

Monotherapy

Aspirin

Aspirin has been studied in primary and secondary prevention of stroke and other vascular events in doses ranging from as low as 30 to as high as 1,500 mg per day. From a pharmacological standpoint, 75 mg per day is enough to block the production of the prothrombotic thromboxane A_2 by inhibiting the enzyme cyclooxygenase virtually completely (see fig. 1). Doses below 50 mg per day make for a less complete blockade but also preserve the production of the antithrombotic prostacyclin. The Antiplatelet Trialists' Collaboration has been performing large meta-analyses of different antiplatelet drugs. In trials comparing different doses of aspirin, ≥75 mg per day was not significantly superior or inferior to <75 mg per day. In studies examining aspirin versus placebo, doses below 75 mg per day were slightly less effective. There was a trend towards the 75–150 mg per day range being most effective in preventing vascular events. In a subset of 21 studies of patients with previous transient ischemic attack (TIA) or stroke, the Antiplatelet Trialists' Collaboration concluded that aspirin reduced the risk of stroke, myocardial infarction, or vascular death from 21.4 to 17.8% over a 2-year period, with an odds reduction of 22% [1]. Risk reductions were similar for men and women, across age groups, and in the presence or absence of diabetes mellitus or elevated blood pressure.

However, aspirin increases the risk of major bleeding by about 70% over placebo, but the absolute annual risk increase is only 0.13%, meaning that about 770 patients have to take aspirin for one year to induce one additional major bleeding incident [2]. Doses >325 mg per day increase this risk, and hence recommended doses are 50–325 mg per day. Because a few days of treatment are required to reach a steady state, loading with doses of 160–300 mg per day is advised. Aspirin cannot be recommended for primary prevention in the general population.

Conditions that may reduce the effectiveness of aspirin include polymorphisms in the gene for cyclooxygenase 1 or other enzymes involved in thromboxane production, increased production of thromboxane in cells other than platelets, high platelet turnover, and concomitant use with other drugs, especially NSAIDS such as ibuprofen and naproxen, which compete for the active center of cyclooxygenase. While poor response to aspirin is related to an increased risk of vascular events and may be overcome by increasing the dose or switching to another agent, there is no direct evidence to support this approach.

Ticlopidine

Ticlopidine is an irreversible inhibitor of the $P2Y_{12}$ receptor. Via this mechanism, it blocks platelet activation through ADP and the glycoprotein IIb/IIIa pathway (see fig. 1). It has been shown to be about as effective in preventing cardiovascular events as aspirin. Because of the preferable safety profile, it has been largely abandoned for its successor, clopidogrel.

Clopidogrel

The standard dose for clopidogrel is 75 mg per day; loading with 300 mg is advised. Most of the evidence on the use of clopidogrel in secondary prevention of vascular events comes from the 1996 CAPRIE trial. Qualifying events for inclusion were a mix of atherosclerotic conditions, such as recent ischemic stroke, myocardial infarction,

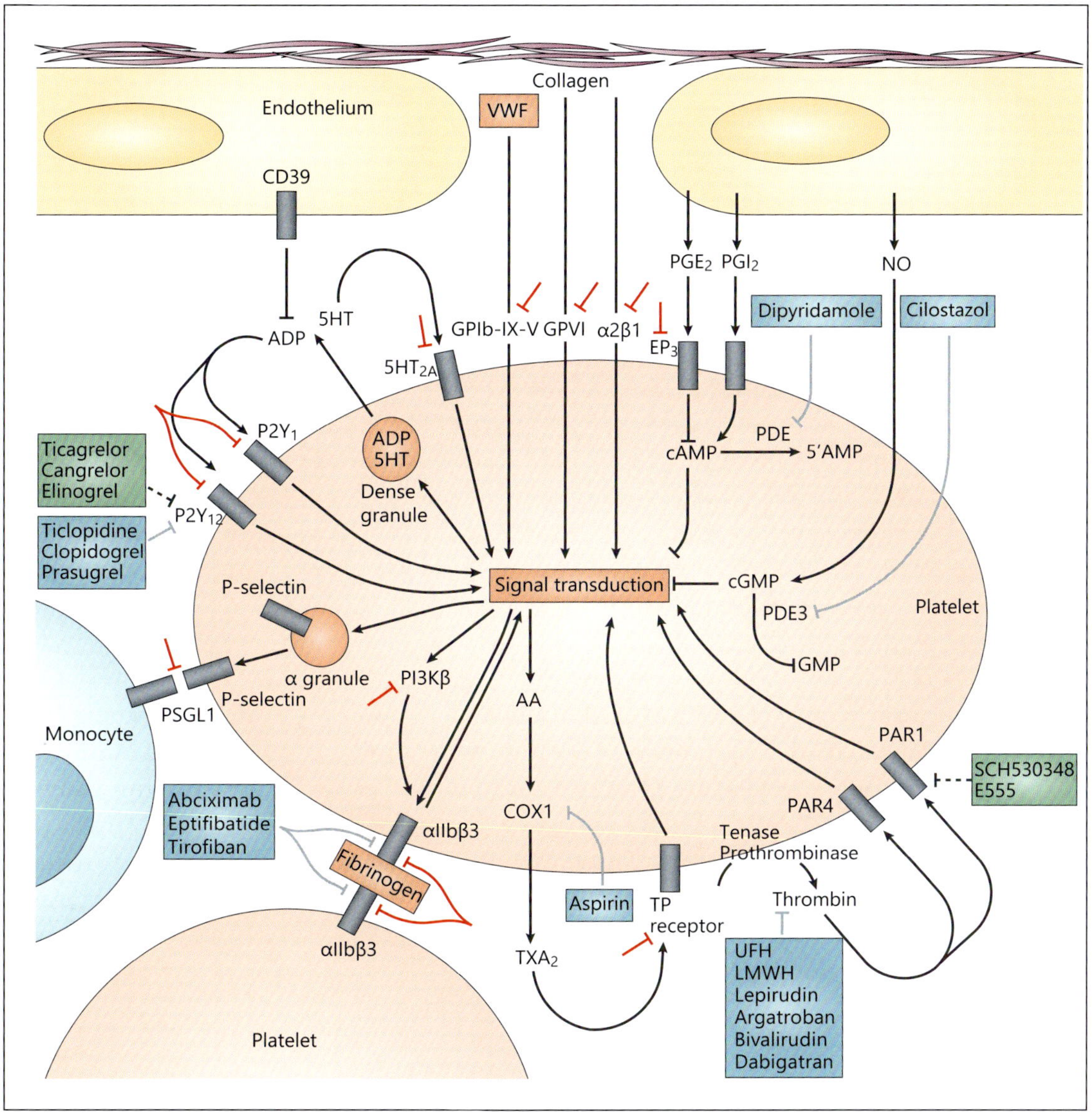

Fig. 1. The complex pathways of platelet activation and molecular targets for antiplatelet agents. Antiplatelet drugs are shown in blue, drugs in clinical development or recently approved are shown in green, investigational strategies are shown in red. AA = Arachidonic acid; COX1 = cyclooxygenase 1; EP_3 = prostaglandin E_2 receptor EP_3 subtype; GPVI = glycoprotein VI; LMWH = low-molecular-weight heparin; NO = nitric oxide; PAR = proteinase-activated receptor; PDE = phosphodiesterase; PG = prostaglandin; PI3Kβ = phosphoinositide 3-kinase β-isoform; PSGL1 = P-selectin glycoprotein ligand 1; TP = thromboxane prostanoid; TXA_2 = thromboxane A_2; UFH = unfractionated heparin; VWF = Von Willebrand factor. Reprinted with permission from Macmillan Publishers Ltd [24].

peripheral artery disease, but not TIA. For all these groups, clopidogrel led to an 8.7% (0.3–16.5) relative risk reduction for a combined end point of ischemic stroke, myocardial infarction, or vascular death compared to aspirin. This treatment effect was, however, not the same among patient groups with similar diseases. While the effect was large and highly significant in the peripheral artery disease group, effects were small and insignificant in patients with ischemic stroke or myocardial infarction as the qualifying events. The efficacy is usually presumed to be similar in TIA and stroke, on the rationale that the two share the same pathophysiology. Bleeding rates were comparable or slightly smaller for clopidogrel [3].

Conditions that may decrease the effect of clopidogrel mainly include concomitant therapy with other drugs or genetic reasons. Clopidogrel is a prodrug, which is transformed to its active metabolite by the cytochrome P system, most notably CYP2C19, CYP3A4/5, CYP2B6, and CYP2C9. Inhibitors of these enzymes may thus decrease the effect of clopidogrel. One such drug is omeprazole (and to a lesser degree other proton pump inhibitors) and should be avoided in these patients. Also, several polymorphisms in the genes to these CYP enzymes have been described, which lead to decreased clopidogrel activation.

Cilostazol

Cilostazol is an agent with a similar mode of action as dipyridamole (see fig. 1). It has been studied in secondary prevention after stroke in 2 RCTs (the CASISP and CSPS II trials), where it was more effective than aspirin in preventing vascular events (RR 0.72, 95% CI: 0.57–0.91) with a lower risk of hemorrhagic stroke (RR 0.26, 95% CI: 0.13–0.55) [4]. The caveat here is that both trials included virtually only Asians who have a higher risk of hemorrhagic stroke and hemorrhagic transformation of ischemic stroke than Caucasians or people of African descent. Transferability of study results may be limited and the drug has not been approved in Europe.

Terutroban

Terutroban is a selective antagonist of the thromboxane A_2 receptor, which was said to share anti-inflammatory and antithrombotic effects in addition to antiplatelet activities. The largest secondary prevention trial after stroke/TIAs in patients with atherothrombotic small and large artery diseases, the PERFORM trial, was prematurely stopped for futility reasons >36 months after recruitment of patients. Terutroban was comparable to aspirin in terms of safety and effectiveness.

Other Agents

Prasugrel and ticagrelor are, like ticlopidine and clopidogrel, inhibitors of the $P2Y_{12}$ receptor (see fig. 1). While they have been approved in patients with different coronary conditions, they have not been studied for secondary prevention after stroke or TIA.

Tirofiban is an inhibitor of the glycoprotein GPIIbIIIA ($\alpha IIB\beta_3$), an important molecule in platelet activation (see fig. 1). Since it has to be given IV, it is not suitable for a long-term therapy in secondary prevention. It has been proposed for use in patients shortly after acute ischemic stroke, especially when they are thought to be at high risk of ischemic stroke progression, such as in patients with stenosis of the basilar artery and in low-flow territories. The phase II SaTIS trial has shown that such an approach is feasible and safe with low rates of hemorrhagic complications, but with a lower 5-month mortality rate in the tirofiban group (OR 4.05, 95% CI: 1.1–14.9) [5]. Unfortunately, a phase III trial with this drug has not been performed.

Abciximab is a monoclonal antibody of GPIIbIIIA. The AbESTT-II trial comparing abciximab and placebo in acute stroke was stopped prematurely because, at 3 months, while mortality and morbidity were similar in the study groups, the bleeding risk was excessively higher in the abciximab group.

Combination Regimens

Aspirin plus Extended-Release Dipyridamole

Dipyridamole has a dual mode of action. It blocks adenosine reuptake and thus leads to vasodilation. This effect is temporary because adenosine receptors are consequently downregulated. Its second mode of action is by blocking phosphodiesterase in platelets, which leads to decreased platelet aggregation. Dipyridamole has been shown to be about as effective as aspirin in preventing vascular events [6]. The ESPS2 and ESPRIT trials gave an indication that the combination of an extended-release formula of dipyridamole and aspirin (usually 200/25 b.i.d.) reduces the risk of vascular events over aspirin alone after stroke or TIA (HR 0.82, 95% CI: 0.74–0.91) [7], but the subsequent large PRoFESS trial failed to confirm superiority over clopidogrel [8]. Since clopidogrel is no more effective than aspirin in preventing recurrent stroke, the question was raised whether the effects seen in these earlier trials were due to the relatively low doses given in the aspirin alone groups (50 mg per day in the ESPS2 trial, 30–325 mg per day in ESPRIT, with 44% receiving only 30 mg per day). More recently, the JASAP trial used an aspirin dose of 81 mg per day, closer to the doses commonly prescribed. This trial failed to show equality of aspirin plus dipyridamole compared to aspirin alone [9]. This might have been due to unexpectedly low event rates and short study duration, but there is no evidence that suggests that results would have differed had the study been larger or longer. In PRoFESS, the bleeding risk was slightly higher for aspirin plus dipyridamole than for clopidogrel (HR 1.15, 95% CI: 1.00–1.32) [8].

Dipyridamole is a vasodilator and may cause headaches in up to 30% of patients, usually within the first days, and up to 10% of patients will discontinue the drug because of this. Due to the lower aspirin dose of 50 mg per day compared to the aspirin doses usually prescribed to patients with coronary disease, its use is sometimes discouraged in these patients.

Aspirin plus Clopidogrel

The combination of aspirin and clopidogrel has been of especial interest. It is widely used in patients with acute coronary syndrome or after stenting. Two large trials studied this combination in secondary prevention after stoke or TIA: CHARISMA and MATCH. The CHARISMA trial compared this combination versus aspirin alone in a broad group at high risk for vascular events due to different conditions (about 25 and 12% had a history of stroke and TIA, respectively) and found only minor, mostly insignificant differences in efficacy and safety [10]. The MATCH trial compared the combination versus clopidogrel alone after recent ischemic stroke or TIA [11]. Here, combination treatment was not significantly more effective than clopidogrel alone (RRR 6.4%, 95% CI: –4.6 to 16.3%), but the risk of life-threatening hemorrhage was increased significantly at 2.6 versus 1.3%. However, both trials had the drawback of including many patients several weeks after the index event, while the risk of recurrent ischemic stroke has already declined from a much higher level immediately after the event. The FASTER trial tried to close this gap by including patients within 24 h and with a limited observation time of 90 days. This trial had to be terminated due to slow recruitment, however. There were no significant differences in rates of ischemic events or hemorrhages, but a small trend was demonstrated towards reduced rates of vascular events in the combination versus aspirin alone groups. In general, the combined therapy of aspirin and clopidogrel cannot be recommended for secondary prevention after stroke and TIA, mainly for safety issues. It remains unclear whether combined treatment initiated immediately after the event and given for a limited time (i.e. no more than 3 months) has a favorable risk/benefit ratio as was shown in trials with cardiovascular patients.

When to Switch

As a matter of drug trial designs and sponsors, the issue of changing drugs in patients who develop (recurrent) vascular events despite antiplatelet therapy has not been investigated. In the absence of significantly different benefit/risk aspects of pharmacodynamically different antiplatelet drugs, current guidelines include staying on the same agent, adding another agent, switching to another antithrombotic agent (usually from aspirin to clopidogrel or to aspirin plus dipyridamole), or switching to anticoagulation (sometimes even without proof of non-valvular atrial fibrillation, NVAF). Therefore, guidelines and experts emphasize the need to carefully reevaluate intermittent NVAF as a possible cause of some previous events in patients who may potentially benefit from anticoagulants.

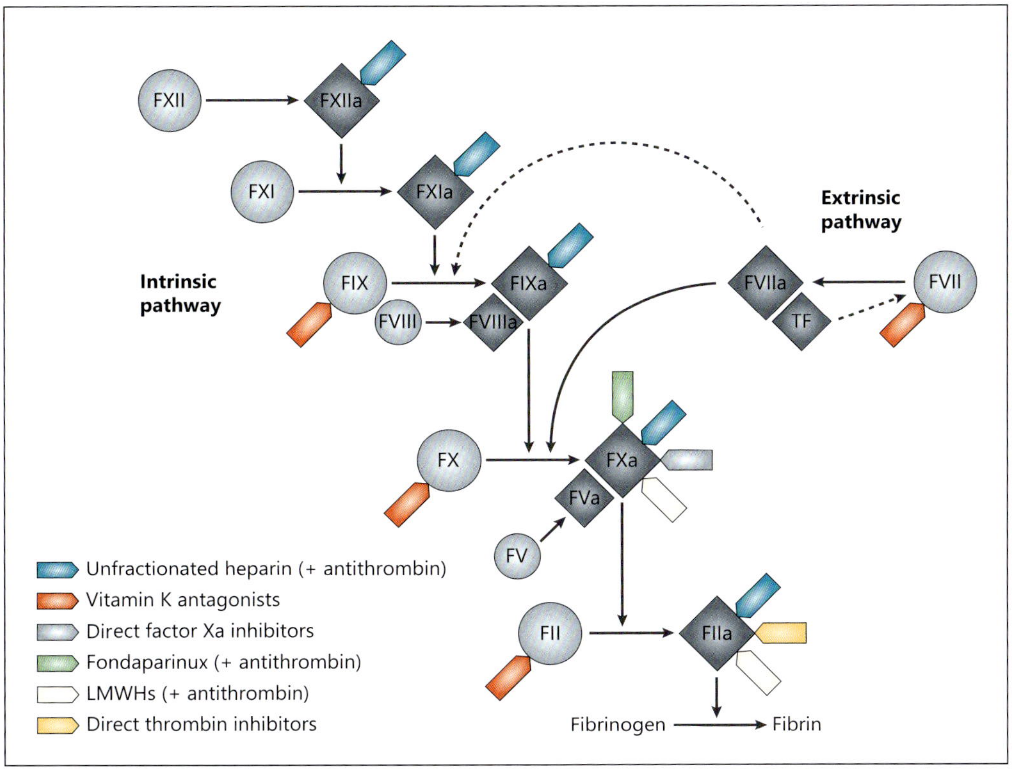

Fig. 2. A simplified schematic of the blood anticoagulation cascade and the targets of different anticoagulants. Factors Xa and IIa (thrombin) are part of the common final pathway of the extrinsic and intrinsic pathways. This makes them good targets for anticoagulants. F = Factor; TF = tissue factor. Reprinted with permission from Macmillan Publishers Ltd [25].

Anticoagulants

Vitamin K Antagonists

Vitamin K antagonists (VKAs) are a class of drugs which inhibit the γ-glutamylcarboxylase in a competitive, dose-dependent and reversible manner. γ-Glutamylcarboxylation is an important step in the synthesis of the coagulation factors II, VII, IX, X, as well as the anticoagulatory proteins C and S (see fig. 2). By this mechanism, these drugs inhibit mostly the intrinsic pathway of coagulation and work as powerful anticoagulants. Their effect can be measured with the prothrombin time (PT) or its standardized derivative, the international normalized ratio (INR). Different levels of anticoagulation have been studied: 'mild' anticoagulation with an INR in about the 1.5–2.0 range, 'medium' anticoagulation (INR 2.0–3.0) and high-intensity anticoagulation (INR 3.0–4.5). Since necessary doses vary widely intra- and interpersonally, therapy monitoring is necessary but may be difficult if a metabolic and drug-associated interaction exists.

Internationally, warfarin is the agent most widely used in clinical practice and studies. Phenprocoumon and acenocoumarol are two other agents of this group used in some countries (such as in Germany), whose main differences are the longer and shorter half-life, respectively.

Historically, VKAs have been used in a variety of conditions in the primary and secondary prevention of stroke and TIA. Over time and as research progressed, few of these conditions are still considered an indication for anticoagulation. Today, the most important indication for warfarin and its likes are atrial fibrillation and venous thrombosis, for which it was the only effective treatment until recently. In NVAF, warfarin reduces the risk of ischemic stroke by 67% (95% CI: 54–77%) compared to placebo and by 37% (95% CI: 23–48%) compared to antiplatelet therapy. The risk of major hemorrhage is increased by about 66% (95% CI: –18 to 235%) compared to control or placebo, but with a low increase in the absolute risk of 0.3% per year. Compared with aspirin, the risk is increased by about 70% (95% CI: –14 to 234%); the increase in absolute risk is 0.2% per year [12]. Today, the recommended target range for the INR is usually 2.0–3.0.

Historically, many physicians have chosen to use warfarin in patients who suffer from cardiac heart failure (usually when the left ventricular ejection fraction, LVEF, was below 30–35%). The rationale for this is the high risk of embolism when a thrombus forms in the left ventricle. Others have chosen a stricter approach and will anticoagulate only when highly reduced LVEF is accompanied by a ventricular aneurysm. Either way, data to support any specific course of action were sparse, of limited quality and contradictory. The WARCEF trial has compared warfarin (INR range of 2.0–3.5) with aspirin 325 mg per day in patients with an LVEF of 35% or less, but no clear indication for either aspirin or warfarin (such as atrial fibrillation) was given. In these patients, a composite outcome of death, ischemic stroke or cerebral hemorrhage was equally common in both groups with rates of 7.47 versus 7.93% per year for warfarin and aspirin, respectively (HR 0.93, 95% CI: 0.79–1.10). However, the rate of ischemic stroke was reduced to 0.72% for warfarin versus 1.36% per year for aspirin (HR 0.52, 95% CI: 0.33–0.82). Major hemorrhages were, on the other hand, more common in the warfarin group, with a rate of 1.78 versus 0.78% per year in the aspirin group (HR 2.05, 95% CI: 1.36–3.12) [13]. With these data, no clear advice on primary stroke prevention in patients with cardiac failure can be given. In the case of secondary prevention in a patient with a recent history of stroke or TIA and cardiac failure, one could argue that the risk of a recurrent ischemic event seems higher than in primary prevention. But here again, good data are sparse, and WARCEF is unlikely to fill the gap because only 12.7% of patients had a history of stroke or TIA. So, in this scenario, the decision should be made individually as well.

Another area hotly debated was whether patients with patent foramen ovale (PFO) should be treated with aspirin, warfarin, or the new contender, interventional closure. Again, good data are scarce and contradictory, however the 1:4 incidence of a PFO in a healthy population and the small risk of stroke recurrence in cryptogenic strokes with PFO underlines the benign nature of PFO without additional (e.g. inflammatory) concomitants; risk moderators commonly named are atrial septum aneurysm, size and shunt volume. The CLOSURE [14], PC [15] and RESPECT [16] trials all failed to establish superiority of device closure over medical therapy, regardless of shunt size or presence of an atrial aneurysm. Also, there was no indication that either of the medical treatments was better than the other or that some patients may benefit more than others. One should keep in mind, however, that these trials began more than ten years ago and has several technical and design problems.

The use of warfarin in atherosclerosis has been studied in several large studies, namely WARSS, WASID and ESPRIT. While, naturally, results differ between studies, there is now little if any indication left for oral anticoagulation on the basis of atherosclerosis. For the case of atherosclerosis of the aortic arch, a dual antiplatelet vs. anticoagulant therapy on top of best medical treatment was studied: unfortunately the ARCH trial stopped randomization due to lack of funding after recruitment of 345 patients (756-1488 were calculated).

Another indication for VKAs is the presence of cardiac implants such as mechanical, artificial heart valves or implantable heart assist devices. INR ranges depend on the type of implant and patient characteristics.

γ-Glutamylcarboxylase is involved in other pathways as well, especially in bone metabolism, which explains why VKAs may cause osteoporosis. Other complications include a hypercoagulatory state early in the treatment, when protein C and S levels decrease, and hepatotoxicity. There are many interactions with other drugs, but also with food: vitamin K is essential in photosynthesis and found in high doses in many green vegetables, especially cabbage and lettuce. Drugs mainly interfere with the hepatic metabolism of warfarin or by displacing it from plasma protein binding. In the case of a severe hemorrhage, the effect of VKAs can be reversed by vitamin K, prothrombin complex concentrate, or fresh frozen plasma.

Novel Anticoagulants

VKAs have not only been the standard, but almost the only choice in long-term anticoagulation. After some failed attempts with new agents, new drugs have recently entered the field with a different mechanism and different safety and efficacy profiles. All of them have been tested against warfarin in the secondary and primary prevention of stroke and TIA in patients with atrial fibrillation as well as in patients with venous thrombosis; one of them (apixaban) has also been tested against aspirin. All of these agents have fewer but different drug interactions than warfarin and far fewer food interactions. All of them are, at least partially, secreted renally, so renal insufficiency is an issue for dosage and contraindication in all of them. They have short half-lives, which is favorable in the case of hemorrhage but requires better adherence by the patient. None of them requires therapeutic monitoring. When trying to monitor, routine tests of coagulation are of limited value and, in the case of relevant hemorrhage, there is currently no well-established procedure to counter the effect of any of these drugs (however, good data are lacking about the risk/benefit strategies in patients presenting with intracerebral hemorrhage while on VKAs, too). While many similarities among novel anticoagulants (NoACs) are present, there are differences as well. These include the characteristics of patients studied, measures of efficacy and safety, approval of different doses by different governing authorities, one having been tested against aspirin, and once- versus twice-daily administration.

Dabigatran

Dabigatran is a direct, competitive and reversible inhibitor of thrombin (factor IIa), the enzyme that converts fibrinogen to fibrin (see fig. 2). The RE-LY trial was designed to prove non-inferiority of dabigatran (either 110 or 150 mg b.i.d.) versus warfarin (INR range 2.0–3.0). In this trial, dabigatran 110 mg b.i.d. was as effective as warfarin in preventing stroke or systemic embolism, while rates of major hemorrhage were lower for this dose. Dabigatran 150 mg b.i.d., on the other hand, was more effective in preventing stroke or embolism with an elevated bleeding risk. All-cause mortality was slightly lower (borderline significant) in the dabigatran 150 mg group than in the warfarin group. In short: dabigatran 110 mg b.i.d. seems to be as efficient as warfarin but safer, while 150 mg b.i.d. is as safe as warfarin but more efficient (for detailed data, see table 1) [17]. A subgroup analysis of only the patients with previous stroke or TIA showed consistent results [18].

Rates of myocardial infarction were slightly elevated in both 110 and 150 mg compared to warfarin. Dyspepsia and discontinuation of study medication were also more common for dabigatran.

There are no known effects of dabigatran on the metabolism of other drugs. Inhibitors or inductors of p-glycoprotein may, however, influence the serum levels of dabigatran. These include some antiarrhythmics. Based on the data from RE-LY, different governing authorities have chosen to approve different doses: the FDA has approved 75 mg b.i.d. for patients with a creatinine clearance of 15–30 ml/min, but has not approved the 110-mg b.i.d. dose. European agencies have, on the other hand, not approved a 75-mg dose but did approve 110 mg b.i.d., especially for patients over the age of 80 years or with a creatinine clearance of 30–50 ml/min. The phase II trial RE-ALIGN studying dabigatran for patients with mechanical heart valves was recently halted due to safety concerns.

Therapy monitoring via PT (PT/INR) is not possible. The activated partial thromboplastin time (aPTT) is another test that is readily available but its results do not correlate well with dabigatran concentrations. Regular thrombin time can be used to determine whether relevant concentrations of dabigatran are present. Calibrated throm-

Table 1. Study parameters

Drug	Dabigatran 110	Dabigatran 150	Rivaroxaban	Apixaban	Apixaban
Trial	RE-LY [17]	RE-LY [17]	ROCKET-AF[1] [19]	AVERROES [19]	ARISTOTLE [21]
Mean patient age, years	71.4	71.5	73	70	70
Mean $CHADS_2$-score	2.1	2.2	3.5	2.0	2.1
Previous TIA/stroke, %	20	20	55	14	19
Mean time in the therapeutic range (TTR, %)	64	64	58	N/A	62
Rate of stroke or systemic embolism, % per year[2]	1.5 vs. 1.69 RR 0.91 (0.74–1.11)	1.11 vs. 1.69 RR 0.66 (0.53–0.82)	1.7 vs. 2.2 HR 0.79 (0.66–0.96)	1.6 vs. 3.7 HR 0.45 (0.32–0.62)	1.27 vs. 1.60 HR 0.79 (0.66–0.95)
Rate of major bleeding, % per year[2]	2.71 vs. 3.36 RR 0.80 (0.69–0.93)	3.11 vs. 3.36 RR 1.16 (1.00–1.34)	3.6 vs. 3.4 HR 1.04 (0.90–1.20)	1.4 vs. 1.2 HR 1.13 (0.74–1.75)	2.13 vs. 3.09 HR 0.69 (0.60–0.80)
Mortality from any cause, % per year[2]	3.75 vs. 4.13 RR 0.91 (0.80–1.03)	3.64 vs. 4.13 RR 0.88 (0.77–1.00)	1.9 vs. 2.2 HR 0.85 (0.70–1.02)	3.5 vs. 4.4 HR 0.79 (0.62–1.02)	3.52 vs. 3.94 HR 0.87 (0.80–0.998)

[1] Per-protocol analysis.
[2] All rates vs. warfarin, except for the AVERROES trial (vs. aspirin). Hazard ratio or relative risk (in the RE-LY trial) and its 95% CI.

bin time and ecarin clotting time correlate better and should be preferred, but are not always available. There is no antidote proven effective against dabigatran. Some authors suggest the use of prothrombin complex concentrate, fresh frozen plasma or recombinant factor VII. Hemodialysis is a possibility, especially in patients with renal insufficiency. Due to its generally short half-life, waiting and administering activated charcoal may be enough in less severe cases.

Direct Oral Factor Xa Inhibitors

These represent another class of NoACs: drugs that inhibit the activated form of factor X, the enzyme that converts prothrombin to thrombin (see fig. 2). They are called direct, because they bind directly to the serine protease at the active center of the target enzyme and do not depend on the presence of antithrombin to act. So far, two drugs have been studied in the prophylaxis of stroke in patients with atrial fibrillation. These are rivaroxaban and apixaban. The first has been approved in many countries including the US and Europe, while the latter has yet to be approved in the US. Other substances of this class are currently under investigation.

Rivaroxaban

Rivaroxaban was the first drug in this class to be approved for the prevention of stroke and systemic embolism in patients with atrial fibrillation. This decision was based on ROCKET-AF, a double-blind, non-inferiority trial comparing rivaroxaban 20 mg once daily (15 mg once daily in patients with a creatinine clearance of 30–49 ml/min) with warfarin with a target INR of 2.0–3.0. The rates of stroke or systemic embolism in the per-protocol analysis were lower for rivaroxaban. Overall, bleeding rates were similar for both drugs while critical and fatal bleeding was less common in the rivaroxaban group. Lastly, there was a trend towards all-cause mortality being lower for rivaroxaban (for detailed data, see table 1) [19].

With the recommended once-daily administration, the half-life of rivaroxaban is about 5–9 h in the younger and 11–13 h in the older population, which usually suggests twice-daily administration. This might be more effective and safe than once daily. On the other hand, administration once daily may improve patient adherence and thus efficacy and safety. When taken, one third is secreted unmetabolized through the kidneys, the rest is metabolized in the liver. Rivaroxaban is a substrate of the cytochrome P450 isoenzymes 3A4 and 2J2 and the p-glycoprotein. Inductors or inhibitors of these enzymes will influence serum levels of rivaroxaban. This is especially the case for CYP3A4 and concerns a number of different drugs and grapefruit juice. It has no known effects on serum levels of other drugs. Therapy monitoring is possible through calibrated anti-factor-Xa assays. PT and aPTT are not reliable. There are no established procedures for the case of major bleeding. Again, some authors suggest the use of prothrombin complex concentrate, fresh frozen plasma or recombinant factor VII. Due to its usually short half-life, waiting and administering activated charcoal may be enough in less severe cases. Hemodialysis is not an option because of the high level of plasma protein binding. A specific antidote (a recombinant, inactive form of factor Xa with retained affinity to the drug) is under development.

Apixaban

Apixaban is the other drug of this group recently approved for stroke prevention in patients with atrial fibrillation. It has been studied in two trials: the AVERROES trial compared it with aspirin and the ARISTOTLE trial with warfarin.

In the double-blind superiority trial AVERROES, patients with atrial fibrillation who had a contraindication to warfarin or were not willing to take it were randomized to receive either aspirin (81–324 mg per day) or apixaban 5 mg b.i.d. (2.5 mg b.i.d. for patients >80 years old, with a body weight of ≤60 kg, or a serum creatinine of 1.5 mg/dl or more). The study was terminated early due to an excess of strokes in the aspirin group. Rates of major bleeding were not significantly different in the two groups, and mortality from any cause was slightly lower in the apixaban group (for detailed data, see table 1) [20].

ARISTOTLE was a double-blind, non-inferiority trial of the same doses of apixaban versus warfarin with a target INR of 2.0–3.0. Rates of stroke or systemic embolism, major bleeding, and mortality were all lower in the apixaban group (for detailed data, see table 1) [21].

Apixaban has pharmacokinetics similar to those of rivaroxaban, so the same caveats about concomitant drug use, therapy monitoring and procedures in major hemorrhages apply. Its rate of renal clearance is lower than that of dabigatran or rivaroxaban, so it may be a preferred choice in patients with renal insufficiency. In Europe, the recommended dose for patients with creatinine clearance between 15 and 29 ml/min is 2.5 mg b.i.d.

Comparing VKAs and NoACs

With four alternatives for the prevention of stroke in atrial fibrillation now available – and probably more to come – one may be at a loss as to which drug to choose for which patient. At first sight, warfarin seems to be out of the running for most patients, but even that is not so clear on closer inspection. All three studies above comparing NoACs with warfarin have been criticized for the moderate quality of warfarin therapy as measured by time in the therapeutic range (TTR) of INR values. These ranged from 55% (ROCKET-AF) to 62% (ARISTOTLE) and 64% (RE-LY), and are all below the recommended value of >70%. Other recent studies with warfarin reported TTR values of 63–74%. As far as has been reported, quality varied considerably between countries and centers, and the advantages of NoACs became less clear and finally vanished for the best centers. Thus, patients on VKAs and with a TTR of ≥75% are not likely to profit from switching, while those with a lower TTR may. One should be careful, however, when this is due to low adherence on the part of the patient: just one missed dose of these drugs may mean insufficient anticoagulation. Warfarin may also be preferable in patients with advanced renal insufficiency as it is almost completely metabolized in the liver. Although between one fifth and one third of patients in these trials were co-medicated with aspirin, the amount of experience is not comparable to co-medication of anti-platelet drugs with warfarin, and it is not generally recommended. There is no information on a triple therapy of NoACs and dual platelet therapy: when necessary, warfarin still remains the drug of choice. Recent studies of NoACs in patients with venous thromboembolism have had similar aspects to them and shown mixed results, suggesting that VKAs may have a larger role in this indication, too [22].

Choosing just among the NoACs is not a simple task, either. There are some obvious differences: rivaroxaban has to be taken only once daily, dabigatran has the option of weighing risks of bleeding versus embolism individually but comes with an increased rate of dyspepsia (and maybe myocardial infarction), and apixaban has been tested against aspirin and may appeal to some patients seeking the 'mild alternative'. Beyond these differences, one is forced to draw one's conclusions from indirect comparisons of these trials. When trying to do so, one should be aware of the following: not only did the study populations differ in terms of stroke risk and previous therapies, but also in the quality of warfarin therapy. Especially this last item introduces an uncontrolled bias. So, with these limitations in mind, Lip et al. [23] concluded that dabigatran 150 mg b.i.d. seems to be superior to rivaroxaban in preventing stroke and systemic embolism, while 110 mg b.i.d. seems to be equally effective. Apixaban seems to be as effective as rivaroxaban or either dose of dabigatran. Major bleeding seemed to be less common for apixaban than rivaroxaban and the higher dose of dabigatran, but about as common as for the lower dose of dabigatran.

References

1 Antithrombotic Trialists' Collaboration: Collaborative meta-analysis of randomised trials of antiplatelet therapy for prevention of death, myocardial infarction, and stroke in high risk patients. BMJ 2002;324:71–86.

2 McQuaid KR, Laine L: Systematic review and meta-analysis of adverse events of low-dose aspirin and clopidogrel in randomized controlled trials. Am J Med 2006;119:624–638.

3 CAPRIE Steering Committee: A randomised, blinded, trial of clopidogrel versus aspirin in patients at risk of ischaemic events (CAPRIE). CAPRIE Steering Committee. Lancet 1996;348:1329–1339.

4 Kamal AK, Naqvi I, Husain MR, Khealani BA: Cilostazol versus aspirin for secondary prevention of vascular events after stroke of arterial origin. Cochrane Database Syst Rev 2011;CD008076.

5 Siebler M, Hennerici MG, Schneider D, Reutern von GM, Seitz RJ, Rother J, et al: Safety of tirofiban in acute ischemic stroke: The SaTIS Trial. Stroke 2011;42:2388–2392.

6 De Schryver EL, Algra A, van Gijn J: Dipyridamole for preventing stroke and other vascular events in patients with vascular disease. Cochrane Database Syst Rev 2003;CD001820.

7 ESPRIT Study Group, Halkes PHA, van Gijn J, Kappelle LJ, Koudstaal PJ, Algra A: Aspirin plus dipyridamole versus aspirin alone after cerebral ischaemia of arterial origin (ESPRIT): randomised controlled trial. Lancet 2006;367:1665–1673.

8 Sacco RL, Diener H-C, Yusuf S, Cotton D, Ôunpuu S, Lawton WA, et al: Aspirin and extended-release dipyridamole versus clopidogrel for recurrent stroke. N Engl J Med 2008;359:1238–1251.

9 Uchiyama S, Ikeda Y, Urano Y, Horie Y, Yamaguchi T: The Japanese Aggrenox (extended-release dipyridamole plus aspirin) stroke prevention versus aspirin programme (JASAP) study: a randomized, double-blind, controlled trial. Cerebrovasc Dis 2011;31:601–613.

10 Bhatt DL, Fox KAA, Hacke W, Berger PB, Black HR, Boden WE, et al: Clopidogrel and aspirin versus aspirin alone for the prevention of atherothrombotic events. N Engl J Med 2006;354:1706–1717.

11 Diener H-C, Bogousslavsky J, Brass LM, Cimminiello C, Csiba L, Kaste M, et al: Aspirin and clopidogrel compared with clopidogrel alone after recent ischaemic stroke or transient ischaemic attack in-high-risk patients (MATCH): randomised, double-blind, placebo-controlled trial. Lancet 2004;364:331–337.

12 Hart RG, Pearce LA, Aguilar MI: Meta-analysis: antithrombotic therapy to prevent stroke in patients who have nonvalvular atrial fibrillation. Ann Intern Med 2007;146:857–867.

13 Homma S, Thompson JLP, Pullicino PM, Levin B, Freudenberger RS, Teerlink JR, et al: Warfarin and aspirin in patients with heart failure and sinus rhythm. N Engl J Med 2012;366:1859–1869.

14 Furlan AJ, Reisman M, Massaro J, Mauri L, Adams H, Albers GW, et al: Closure or medical therapy for cryptogenic stroke with patent foramen ovale. N Engl J Med 2012;366:991–999.

15 Meier B, Kalesan B, Mattle HP, Khattab AA, Hildick-Smith D, Dudek D, et al: Percutaneous closure of patent foramen ovale in cryptogenic embolism. N Engl J Med 2013;368:1083–1091.

16 Carroll JD, Saver JL, Thaler DE, Smalling RW, Berry S, MacDonald LA, et al: Closure of patent foramen ovale versus medical therapy after cryptogenic stroke. N Engl J Med 2013;368:1092–1100.

17 Connolly SJ, Ezekowitz MD, Yusuf S, Eikelboom J, Oldgren J, Parekh A, et al: Dabigatran versus warfarin in patients with atrial fibrillation. N Engl J Med 2009;361:1139–1151.

18 Diener H-C, Connolly SJ, Ezekowitz MD, Wallentin L, Reilly PA, Yang S, et al: Dabigatran compared with warfarin in patients with atrial fibrillation and previous transient ischaemic attack or stroke: a subgroup analysis of the RE-LY trial. Lancet Neurology 2010;9:1157–1163.

19 Patel MR, Mahaffey KW, Garg J, Pan G, Singer DE, Hacke W, et al: Rivaroxaban versus warfarin in nonvalvular atrial fibrillation. N Engl J Med 2011;365:883–891.
20 Connolly SJ, Eikelboom J, Joyner C, Diener H-C, Hart R, Golitsyn S, et al: Apixaban in patients with atrial fibrillation. N Engl J Med 2011;364:806–817.
21 Granger CB, Alexander JH, McMurray JJV, Lopes RD, Hylek EM, Hanna M, et al: Apixaban versus warfarin in patients with atrial fibrillation. N Engl J Med 2011;365:981–992.
22 Connors JM: Extended treatment of venous thromboembolism. N Engl J Med 2013;368:767–769.
23 Lip GYH, Larsen TB, Skjøth F, Rasmussen LH: Indirect comparisons of new oral anticoagulant drugs for efficacy and safety when used for stroke prevention in atrial fibrillation. J Am Coll Cardiol 2012;60:738–746.
24 Michelson AD: Antiplatelet therapies for the treatment of cardiovascular disease. Nat Rev Drug Discov 2010;9:154–169.
25 Perzborn E, Roehrig S, Straub A, Kubitza D, Misselwitz F: The discovery and development of rivaroxaban, an oral, direct factor Xa inhibitor. Nat Rev Drug Discov 2011;10:61–75.

Dr. Valentin E. Held
Department of Neurology, UniversitätsMedizin Mannheim
University of Heidelberg
Theodor-Kutzer-Ufer 1–3
DE–68137 Mannheim (Germany)
E-Mail held@neuro.ma.uni-heidelberg.de

Author Index

Subject Index